A CAREGIVER'S JOURNEY
FROM DESPERATION TO HOPE

112 Days

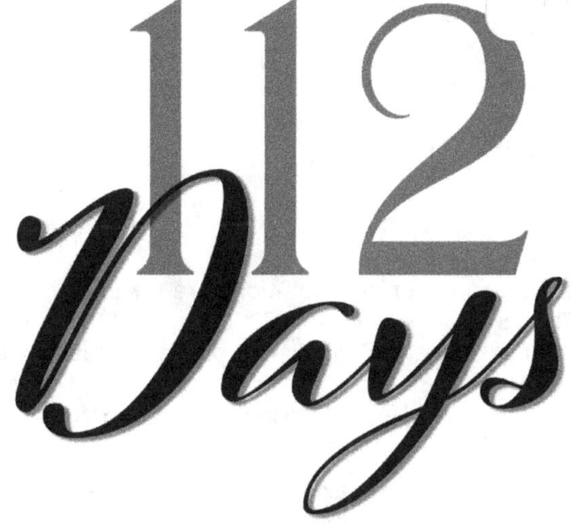

Lauri Smith

112 *Days*

A CAREGIVER'S JOURNEY FROM DESPERATION TO HOPE
© 2023 LAURI SMITH

Published by Lauri Smith | Baytown, Texas

ISBN (Print): 979-88759523-8-8

Printed in the United States of America

Prepared for Publication: www.wendykwalters.com

To contact the author:
l a u r i a s m i t h . c o m

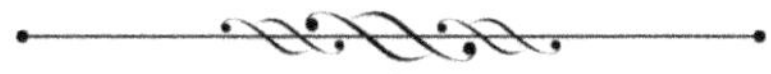

Dedication

This book is dedicated with compassion and empathy to all past, present, and future caregivers. May this be a tool to spread glimpses of hope far and wide and affirm that you are not alone; instead, you are seen, appreciated, and loved.

Disclaimer

This book is a memoir of a specific, intense, stressful season in the author's life. It reflects her present recollections of experiences over time, and it is enhanced by actual journal entries as she served her father as his caregiver. Some events have been compressed, and some dialogue has been recreated.

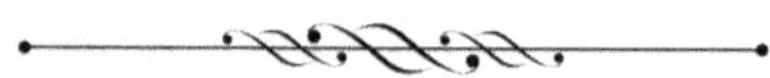

Praise for 112 Days

As a loved one approaches the end of life, will you respond by stepping into a caregiving role? Are you already there? Have you fulfilled this need in the past? Will you consider this in a future scenario that will be here before you know it?

Lauri's book takes you on a journey that is real, painful, and impactful. It is filled with her personal insights and experiences that can help bring direction to your questions and decisions as you seek to care for your loved one as well as yourself. You will come away from reading this book feeling affirmed that you are NOT the first or only human to have to face this difficult time. Lauri's story will take you from desperation to hope in thirteen chapters with dignity and grace.

—JUDY K. KUYKENDALL
Event Coordinator, Caregiver, Friend

112 Days immediately drew me in with the author's raw honesty. As she tells the story of her caregiving experience with her father through the dementia journey and, ultimately, hospice care, I thought of so many patients and families I have worked with over the years. This book is a great resource that I would recommend to anyone with aging loved ones, including those family members/friends who have stepped into the role of caregiver. Medical professionals will also greatly benefit as they will better understand the challenges faced by their patients and those who lovingly care for them.

—NICHOLE HOLMES
LMSW, Hospice Social Worker

In Lauri's achingly honest description of *112 Days*, she shares her experience as a caregiver for her dementia-stricken dad. She pulls back the curtain on a dark experience and shares her journey with us. As a devout Christian, she seeks to find the Light in her purpose, all the while battling feelings of helplessness, hopelessness, and depression. Did God even see her or hear her desperate prayers?

Walk alongside Lauri as she faces God head-on with her questions, as she meets the battles of each day, and as she learns that God is always there, working in the darkness and preparing her to write this much-needed book to be a beacon to anyone who ever has or ever might be a caregiver to a loved one. You will gain knowledge about what she wishes she would have known, and you will learn how God is always by your side—even in the darkness.

—CINDY HIGHTOWER
Friend

Working with Lauri on this manuscript brought up memories of my grandmother's final days—watching her leave us slowly, swept into a world in which we could not join her because of dementia and Alzheimer's. As we were coming to the close of this project, my husband's mother entered hospice, and Lauri's final chapters were timely and spoke directly to our situation with the kind of encouragement and understanding that can come only from someone who has walked where you have trod.

For all who must walk this path and become a caregiver for someone you love, *112 Days* will breathe hope into your spirit and offer comfort to your weary soul. You are not alone, and knowing this is more powerful than you can possibly believe.

—WENDY K. WALTERS
Author, Editor, Motivational Speaker

Contents

You Are Cordially Invited ...

You take a trip to the mailbox on a day much like any other. You open it to find the usual assortment of notices, bills, and junk mail. But wait ... hmmm. What's this?

Open it.

Come on, you know you want to.

It's an invitation—of sorts—from me. This invitation is unique in that it is not to a fun party but to a caregiving life experience. I share my story to help you in your own caregiving journey, either now or in the future. Or perhaps you will never have to walk this particular path, but you have struggles in your life, so I feel sure you can relate.

This book does not contain a brilliant formula for success. It also does not include a promise to make the path you are forging easier.

Well then, why read it?

I'm glad you asked. I hope and pray that as you journey through these pages with me, you will glean some helpful knowledge and, through my experiences, see how God can and will work through literally anyone and bring beauty from anything. God is compassionate, and He does not shy away from desperation, fear, and unfiltered heart cries. God draws nearest in those moments and encourages us to come before Him as we are.

I'll warn you that I lay myself bare here, and it's not pretty. Sometimes it's dark; in fact, it's pretty messy the whole way through. But it's my heart, transparently offered to you in hopes that you will be uplifted by reading about this season that impacted me so deeply I'll never be the same.

255 days.

That's how much I cover in the first chapter of this book: October 1, 2020 – June 13, 2021. These 255 days were preparation for a journey I didn't know I was training for. Oh, there is so much I wish I had known ...

112 days.

The remaining chapters cover the 112 days that changed my life: June 14 – October 3, 2021. These days, though short on the calendar—a brief moment in history—were an eternity lived out. Those 112 days felt like forever, like living underwater with no possibility of coming up for air. It felt like the weight of the water pressing in and the lack of oxygen were a permanent reality.

I had no idea what the world of caregiving for a loved one was all about—the excruciating care decisions to be made, dealing with dementia and bearing the brunt of my father's confusion and frustration, handling hospice, and living with the stress and isolation. I did not know what a gift journaling would be or the comfort of a therapy cat and safe friends to vent to. Above all, as I look back, what stands out most is the grace and love of my God, who walked with me even when I didn't see or feel His presence at all. God ministered to me and nurtured me with His love and grace even when I was unaware.

Whatever situations you are facing in your life right now, I pray my experience will give you hope to cling to and bring a comforting light when your soul feels dark.

—Lauri Smith

June 2023

ENCOURAGEMENT FROM THE LORD

"Lord, you light my lamp;
my God illuminates
my darkness."

PSALM 18:28, CSB

CHAPTER ONE

Realizations of Aging

255 DAYS AND COUNTING TOWARD CAREGIVING

A realization can be like a streak of lightning—brilliant and illuminating. But I have learned that a realization can also be much more subtle and multifaceted, like a tiny flame that grows gradually as more and more is revealed.

My daddy was aging. I suppose I began seeing the signs a few years before his death, but at first, I reasoned them away. Perhaps the little girl in me still thought my daddy was supposed to be strong and healthy. Invincible. But after doing amazingly well for so long, he began to show symptoms that gradually increased.

The first concerning aging symptom I remember was discovered during a 2019 hospital stay. Dad informed the nurse, who was asking all the usual questions, that he had stopped taking his blood thinner medication. He then informed her that his cardiologist had told him he didn't need it. I knew that could not be true because it made no sense. We had a discussion after we were home.

"Dad, I know what you told the nurse is not true, so why did you really stop taking your blood thinner medication?" I asked.

"I don't need it. I don't like taking all those pills," he answered.

"But Dad," I reminded him, "just like the cardiologist on call told you at the hospital, if you don't take this medication, you could have a stroke. That is a great risk! It's life-threatening!"

"I know that. But the right consistency of your blood is an individual thing, and I know my blood is fine, so I don't need the blood thinner," he shot back.

Then it dawned on me that if he had stopped this pill, it was entirely possible he had stopped other medications. "Dad," I asked, "what about your other pills?"

He replied, "I don't take anything anymore. I just decided I was tired of taking all these medications." And he said this in a tone that was almost like he was bragging about it. He was proud of this decision.

"But Dad, you know that taking all your medications at the right time is really important. There is a good reason that you need each one, or they would not have been prescribed. Skipping doses can set you back. You want to be well, don't you?" I appealed to his desire for strength.

He let out a big sigh but told me, "Okay, you're right. I'll take them. I'll start back on them tomorrow."

Relieved, I thought he had gotten the wake-up call he needed to stay on his medications. That turned out not to be the case.

I noticed a few other "normal" aging symptoms. Sometimes he was forgetful, and sometimes he repeated himself, but these things I took in stride. I didn't think of them as degenerative symptoms or signs for alarm. Older people do that, right? Then, as he grew less physically stable, he began using a cane. I wasn't in denial, I knew he was getting older, but I truly believed this was a gradual progression and would continue at the same pace—slow and easy to navigate and address. Why did I think this? I have no idea. Maybe it was just wishful thinking that I chose to believe.

But then, COVID-19 changed the world. In the spring of 2020, required shutdowns and precautions resulted in isolation, which was especially difficult for the elderly. I believe that these circumstances helped a measured progression become increasingly escalated. His aging symptoms began to multiply.

And multiply again.

I started running his errands when the pandemic precautions started in March to help him stay safe, and within a few months, I noticed that he could no longer remember what groceries he needed. Where he used to give me a list each week, he could not remember to make a list. I also noticed that he was not cleaning his home consistently, and he was allowing clutter to pile up more and more. In addition, at some point, he stopped eating frozen leftovers at his home from meals I cooked him. I had done this off and on for years after my mom passed away in 2006, but now instead of eating my leftovers, he became obsessed with eating Banquet pot pies for dinner. This was his dinner choice every single day unless I brought him food and ate with him. He limited his choices for breakfast and lunch too. I know now that this adherence to eating the same things over and over was one of his attempts to control his world as his dementia symptoms increased. I didn't understand this behavior at the time, though, and it was unsettling. As the months progressed, he began eating significantly less and started losing weight noticeably. When I expressed concern, he would say, "I'm eating less because I'm less active. I don't need as much. I'm fine."

I didn't believe him.

In October 2020, my 255-day countdown began; I just didn't know that yet.

I decided to spend more time with him at his home in the evenings after work and on the weekends. I suspected I needed to take a more hands-on approach to see more of what was happening. It was then that I began to get a rough idea of what his daily life was becoming. By this time, he had stopped cleaning his home completely, and the results of eating less became more obvious. His doctor called me after he saw him in November and told me he had lost 23 pounds since his previous appointment in February. Dad adamantly denied that he was depressed, but I feel sure he was, and his doctor agreed and said that normally he would suggest an anti-depressant in this situation. But by now, I had given up nagging him about taking his medications because he had gotten to the point after stopping and starting back several times that he flatly refused them altogether. I could not make him comply, so I knew an anti-depressant medication was out of the question, and his doctor felt the same way. Dad also refused to allow his doctor to run tests because of the concerning weight loss. I tried several times over these months to talk to him about not eating enough, but it was useless. I came to realize that not taking medications and eating less were his choices, and I could not force him to take steps to help improve his health. His doctor agreed.

Bottom line—there was no way to help him see that his mindset was incorrect on anything. Believe me, I tried. Over time, I learned to give up and accept.

He was now becoming more easily confused and flustered. For example, when Dad went to the doctor in November, the doctor prescribed an antibiotic and an over-the-counter probiotic. The pharmacy called to let him know his prescription was ready, and he went to pick it up. He came home and then called me, completely confused.

He was so agitated that I came right over. When I walked in, he had the slip of paper in his hand from the doctor with the name of the probiotic on it, and he thought—no, he insisted—that the name on this paper was the prescription name. He was convinced the pharmacy had given him the wrong medication and was very upset about it. It took me literally about an hour to convince him that he had the correct prescription medication and the other drug listed on the piece of paper was an over-the-counter probiotic.

So yes, by the fall of 2020, there were aging symptoms concerning me, and they were escalating, but I didn't think a complete change in his years-long independent way of living was needed just yet. But then, a few months later, around the beginning of 2021, it became so obvious that I had no choice but to identify a piercing glimpse of what was to come and wonder how long my dad could continue to live alone.

The aging signs were right in front of me for a while, but they had to slap me in the face before I began to see more clearly. I wish it were different, but this is how it happened for me. I suppose that for a time, I saw what I wanted to see and believed Dad when he insisted all was well.

I wanted all to be well. I needed it to be well. It was hard to admit it wasn't.

I wrote the following impressions as though they were coming from him:

1/17/21 Journal Entry—

How must it feel to begin to lose your grasp
on all you have not had to consciously hold to
all your life because it was just always there?

It's all Foggy. Hazy. Blurry.

A distorted perception.

Of everything

Everything that is now skewed and chaotic
and disarrayed.

Nothing is as it should be, but

Everything is normal because it has to be.

Dark.

Lost.

Afraid.

Can't find

Whatever I'm trying to find.

But it's alright. It's all okay.

Because nothing is okay, and that's familiar.

And familiar is safe and good and right.

All, everything,

Is huge and overwhelming and scary ...

So I'll just sit right here in this tiny pinprick of light and order my little bitty world with what I can hold fast to.

I can only hold a very few things, though, so I let go of all the rest, and it all goes away.

I don't need the rest anyway, never did, really.

There.

Now I'm good and safe and free

Until I have to move

At all.

Moving from my precarious position near that tiny light upsets everything because all I hold to shifts and runs through my fingers like sand.

It's so hard to pick grains of sand back up, but I'm forced to pick up one grain at a time because to do any more is way too hard.

Holding tenaciously to my independence, yet wanting help because the world is so much bigger than it used to be. I want help, but only on my terms. And my terms are irrational and illogical. My rationale is irrational. I know this. Yet I don't know this because everything is fine.

Yes, I'm fine. Everything is fine, even if it isn't.

This is how I live. This is my existence.

How on earth did I not see this coming? The signs were all there, in neon colors and big block letters. Well, here's the thing—a gradual progression of anything is sneaky.

And that's how I feel about this—it snuck up on me. Caught me by surprise. I talked to Dad on the phone every single day for years and saw him occasionally until I stepped that up to more frequent visits. Yes, I noticed forgetfulness, which wasn't alarming to me because, after all, he was getting older. And yes, I even suspected dementia, but I didn't have a clue what that even really meant. I equated dementia with forgetfulness. Oh, clueless me. By October 2020, I began to get more concerned, but as his symptoms continued to

> A gradual progression of anything is sneaky.

escalate, it got to a point a few months later that my eyes were forced open to see how he was really living.

By the beginning of 2021, not only had my father ceased cleaning his house, but he had also stopped throwing things away. He gathered items on his kitchen table and counter to throw away, but he just kept adding to the piles. Initially, I would offer to throw things away for him, and he would insist he would do it, but he wouldn't. I was caught between a rock and a hard place of not infringing upon his independence while at the same time beginning to realize that he was following through less and less on daily tasks. Knowing when to step in and when to step back was harder than I ever imagined.

> Knowing when to step in and when to step back was harder than I ever imagined.

One evening, I stopped on the way home from work, grabbed some dinner for us, went by his house, and ate with him. In his pile on the table were food items left over from Meals on Wheels lunches that he had told me several times he was going to throw away. I glanced over there at the pile as I was eating, and there was mold on the apples and oranges. Ugh. So that did it. I arrived the next evening with a garbage bag and got rid of everything on the table and counters in the kitchen that needed to be disposed of.

He was very appreciative when I did this the first time, but his attitude changed as I kept throwing away things for him every time I went over there because I didn't want it to pile up again. If anything went missing, he insisted I had thrown it away. I would typically find whatever he was looking for somewhere other than where he swore it was before I supposedly carelessly got rid of it.

Dementia fractured his ability to trust me. And as he lost his independence, he directed his frustration with that reality toward me more and more.

It hurt.

I also tried working with him to hire someone to clean his house. That did not work out because he refused to pay the cost, so I began cleaning his home myself, but I was very limited in what he would allow me to do. Therefore, for the most part, his home was dusty, dingy, dark, and just … oppressive. And there was clutter everywhere. Papers. Magazines. Junk mail that he thought might be important. He would not allow me to go through any of this clutter, and it just kept increasing.

"Dad," I tried several times to explain, "not having a clean home is not healthy for you. This dust everywhere is not good. Can't you see this? "

Each time he responded, "It doesn't bother me at all! I'm fine, dear. I'm fine!"

He was far from fine, but there was no way to convince him otherwise.

Whenever I expressed concern about anything, and I expressed concern often, he was adamant in his reply, "I'm fine!"

And then, there was the infamous Winter Storm Uri, which blasted Texas in February 2021. I learned the hard way that adding stress and unfamiliar experiences to dementia ramps up all the symptoms to incredible levels. The unusually frigid cold for Texas with snow and ice and wind resulted in many Texans losing power for an extended period. I had a generator hooked up to a charger, but the charger failed, and the generator would not start. Dad and I had no power or heat in either of our homes. One of my wonderful cousins called to check on us and then researched online extensively and found a hotel room, but Dad refused to leave his home, and I could not leave him. Instead, we dressed in layers and piled on blankets as the temperature in his home dropped below 55 degrees during the day and who knows how much colder at night. We had food and water and battery-powered lanterns but no heat. That is, until I *finally* allowed Dad to have his way after he kept on and on and on ... and on, and on, and on, about his ancient Coleman cookstove that was out on his patio, powered by propane. He wore me down. I brought it inside, and we ran the hose to the propane tank through a window. He would not allow me to leave the window unobstructed for some ventilation. Nope, I had to stuff towels in the opening because the cold air was coming in. I was screaming in terror inside myself about how we were going to die of carbon monoxide poisoning. I couldn't say anything of course, so after the burners were lit, I discreetly texted Christian sister friends to pray. Dad kept insisting that we would be fine, and by the grace of God, we were.

Before the power came back on consistently (we had rolling blackouts for days), Dad and I had several discussions about what we would do when the power returned. We agreed that the first priority was making sure his water pipes were good in the attic. His outside pipes were wrapped, and I was dripping all his faucets inside and out, but this cold was worse than we had ever seen, with the wind chill plummeting near zero—unheard of here! We agreed—several times—that I would go up into the attic and check the pipes. Dad would direct me from below where to look, as I had never done this before. So once the power came back on and it appeared it was on to stay this time, I asked him about checking in the attic, and he acted like he had no idea what I was talking about.

"Dad," I reminded him, "remember we had decided we would check in the attic once the power was back to see if your water pipes were okay?"

He looked at me puzzled, with no recollection.

"We agreed that I would go up there, and you would direct me where to look from down here. Remember?"

"My pipes are fine," he insisted. "There is no need to go into the attic; what are you talking about? You are not going up there!"

WHAT??? I thought. And now I found myself watching the ceiling, thinking that at any moment, I would see evidence that water was pouring out in the attic. Praise God this did not happen. Another miracle, as many people in our area had this to deal with when power returned.

Winter Storm Uri with my dad was crazy-making on steroids. I can look back now and see that this was just a little precurser for the caregiving journey I would be embarking on a few months later.

After Uri, my usual routine returned. It took some time for my super-high anxiety level to come back down to normal, but I had to keep going. I kept doing all I could for him while working full time, I spent as much time with him as I could, and I worried. A lot. My stress level kept building, and the fear of the great unknown kept growing. I knew that soon I would need to step up to start a new chapter of my life and his, but I had no idea of the specifics of this chapter. I felt so ill-prepared, and I didn't have a clue what to prepare for. I felt like I was drowning, when really, I wasn't even in the water yet.

> I felt like I was drowning, when really, I wasn't even in the water yet.

Realizations of Aging

Below, I share what I wrote about a month before I began living through the hardest season of my life thus far. Reading this now is a bit chilling. Why? Because it was prophetic. It was so spot on for what I was about to endure; yet, I had no idea when I penned the words.

5/9/21 Journal Entry—

It's deep and dark and cavernous and scary and tumultuous and loud and eerily silent. I am trying to breathe because I know that's important, but I can't draw a breath to literally save my life. And I can't get my bearings at all. I have no idea which way is up, where true north is, or any other direction for that matter. All the guideposts are gone. Everything I know is gone. Everywhere I look becomes nowhere, another dead end.

I'm going to drown. This is it. I can feel it throughout my entire body and down within, all the way to the very core of my being.

But wait. I have a job to do. A very important job, a calling if you will, a season of life thing where IT'S MY TURN.

This is my time to give back. My time to honor another by sacrificing whatever it takes to help him. I'm drowning, but I'm the one who is supposed to be saving him. Yes, from drowning.

Inept does not even begin to describe all I lack to come through to help, even when help is not wanted. And in his world, not only not wanted, but not needed. An insult. Evidence that I do not believe everything is fine when it is. But it's not. A perfect storm blindness brought about by ever-escalating dysfunction of all that makes sense.

Nothing makes sense. So I'm drowning when I am supposed to be the rescuer. I'm dutifully trying to rescue, while at the same time flailing about and struggling to breathe as I'm drowning. I can see how this seems to be destined for colossal failure, with high marks for definite.

A life raft would be very helpful about now. But there is nothing and no one.

But there is. I know it, with a knowing that pierces clean through everything when

I call it to mind. I can sense this even when I can't do anything else. There is a hand to grab onto. But I can't see it, what with all the madness viciously spinning while I'm in the middle of it being tossed about by all the motion that just keeps going faster and faster.

Help me, Jesus, to reach up and trust that You are here to lift me. I must reach up when I have no concept of direction or tangible affirmation. I must reach into nothingness for nothingness to become everythingness. You are all I need and so much more. But the reaching, it must come first. Help me, Jesus.

It was also around this time that I first figured out that Dad was having swallowing issues, another symptom of dementia. He had COPD for years due to asbestos exposure from working at a plant for a long time. Sometimes when he ate, he would cough. So when this symptom of coughing when eating increased, I thought at first that his COPD had worsened. But one evening in May 2021, I had dinner with him and witnessed him obviously struggling to swallow and coughing. It scared me to death, and I did some online research which only increased my fear because it talked about the high risk of asphyxiation, pneumonia, and even death. I tried to talk to him about it, but he denied he was having any trouble swallowing. He had no idea why I thought that. Sometimes this issue was better than others with no pattern, and down the road, this was not an urgent health concern compared to the ongoing weight loss. But it was scary to witness.

Another new symptom that I began to notice around this time was that he was no longer washing clothes, and he was wearing the same clothes over and over. I wanted to start doing his laundry for him, but he would not allow me to. He said he would do it, but by this time, I knew he wouldn't, just like he wouldn't clean the house.

I also realized that his personal hygiene care had diminished. I noticed he had stopped showering every evening like he had done all my life. We talked about it. I tried encouraging him to shower by telling him how much better he would feel if he was clean. We also talked about the physical makeup of his shower and whether he felt safe because I thought just maybe he was afraid he would fall in the shower. Nope. He showed me how his shower was a custom set up by the previous owners of his house, and it was safe with things to grab hold of if he felt unsteady. He insisted he felt safe. I offered to be with him right outside the door when he showered, and he insisted that was unnecessary. The first few times I brought this up, he would say he would shower the next day, but he never did. He finally told me he didn't take showers because he didn't think it was important anymore, another sign of depression and dementia.

Forcing him to shower was not an option. I did not have the physical strength, but I also was not emotionally or mentally in a place to assert authority to override his decision. Sadly, he didn't shower anymore for the rest of his life. Even when hospice care started, and he could have had someone come and help him shower or bathe, he refused. He told me repeatedly that he took "spit baths," and maybe for a time, he did, but not for long.

I hated seeing him like this. He had always been strong, independent, and reliable. Now he was sad, angry, and difficult. I kept trying to remember who he had been, not who he was right now. But even the remembrance gave me no comfort.

He was declining faster and faster, like a snowball flying down a mountain—growing and spinning more and more as the incline moved toward vertical.

And I was the one at the bottom trying to climb the vertical incline to help slow his descent and navigate the way down. He was a snowball flying, and I was slowly climbing up. He left me behind in a flash—staring after him in horror as he plummeted beneath me. I found myself constantly changing my position, trying to get close to him to help, over and over and over. Repeatedly seeing only futility.

But I kept trying.

I had no other choice.

ENCOURAGEMENT FROM THE LORD

"When you go through deep waters,
I will be with you.

When you go through rivers of
difficulty, you will not drown.

When you walk through the fire of
oppression, you will not be burned up;
the flames will not consume you."

ISAIAH 43:2, NLT

CHAPTER TWO

The Beginning of Forever

AND SO IT BEGINS ...

I wrote the following paragraph in my journal early in the morning of my first day as Dad's caregiver before I headed to his house to begin this new season:

6/14/21 Early Morning Journal Entry—

And so it begins. A new journey.

Dad and I talked last night, and I am going to be his caregiver. He was so relieved when I offered. He is just not comfortable with anyone else. I'm terrified and feel very inadequate for this and very alone. But all that is lies, and I know the truth. God's got this. I'm not alone because He is with me, and He will equip me.

Yes, I confidently said that God would equip me to handle this because I felt I should do it. I felt like God was leading me to be Dad's caregiver. And I knew it was the right thing to do. It was what any caring person should do for their parent if they had the opportunity and the relationship was safe. That makes sense, right? I felt that I was being obedient to God to do this, so surely He would equip me to do it. "He doesn't call the equipped; He equips the called." I've heard that well-known saying for years, and I completely believed it.

But that's not what happened in this season. I was never equipped with anything to forge this new path. Instead, I was thrust into a new, unfamiliar location with no tools or knowledge. The "equipping" I experienced revealed what sheer desperation looked like and what it meant to rely on God completely even though I felt alone. I know now that this strange and painful type of equipping was necessary and orchestrated by my good God, but it surely didn't feel good at the time.

This first day of caregiving began with me fixing Dad some breakfast. I immediately noticed that he was coughing and struggling to swallow, and his breakfast was just cereal and toast and jam. To explain why he was coughing, Dad accused me of putting too much jam on his toast. *Really?* I thought.

This is how the day started. Bumpy but not impossible. Then it got worse. Much worse.

I was so unprepared when I embarked on this caregiving journey. When I talked with Dad the evening before and agreed to be his caregiver, I envisioned staying with him several hours a day and working from home several hours too. I thought of it as being with him part-time and working part-time, going back and forth between our homes that were two streets apart. I planned on fixing him breakfast, lunch, and dinner each day, staying with him for a time after each meal and cleaning up, then going home to work and coming back for the next meal with him. In my mind, this routine was doable, so that was my plan in my dream world that I was still living in.

Until ...

I left Dad's later that morning to run a couple of errands for him while he was napping, and I made what I thought was an important and helpful phone call while I was out to clarify some text message communication and ensure I was on the same page with the recipient.

"Ms. Smith," the woman said, "based on our initial assessment of your dad and from the information you have provided me by text, we are concerned your father should not be left alone—at all."

Did you hear that loud crash?

That was my wonderful workable plan falling apart during a phone conversation with the owner of the hospice company that had just started the process of home hospice with Dad. She rocked my world until everything shook and trembled and came down in chaotic scattered pieces all around me. "What do you mean he shouldn't be left alone *at all*?" I asked, not quite comprehending what that meant for him or for me. You see, I thought we were a team—the hospice company and me—so I had diligently tried to fill her in on all the signs of decline I saw and my concerns. In my mind, what I shared with her had all been little things, nothing major. I was just giving her an FYI to help keep them informed and find out what I should be on the lookout for. She completely turned that around.

"Well, from our assessment and from what you told me, I don't think being left alone is in your dad's best interest. But the choice, of course, is completely up to you," she offered. In other words, "This is all on you."

To me, it felt like she used my openness against me. I had shared with her honestly, holding nothing back because I believed they were there to support me as I supported my dad. But the more she talked, the more I realized I was on my own.

While she agreed with me that there were levels of dementia, she would not give me any indication of how severe she felt Dad's dementia was at that point. Instead, she said, "You are his 'essential caregiver,' so all decisions about your father's care are fully yours to make. We do not advise you on what to do or how to respond to his symptoms. That isn't our role. All patients react differently in this season of their life, and we are not experts. You are the expert on your dad's care."

I thought they would reassure me. I thought I would find their support and encouragement comforting as they shared insights from their expertise. This conversation made it clear that this was not to be the case, so I started scrambling. I tried to wrap my mind around what all this completely unexpected information meant:

- Hospice would make no recommendations or suggestions.

- Hospice would not share any knowledge they had gained from medical experience with aging patients.

- Right or wrong, I gathered that I should expect nothing from hospice care beyond checking his vitals twice a week and noting anything of concern.

I was stunned. This was just day one!

Every bit of how to handle all the twists and turns of this new season was up to me, and I had absolutely no idea what I was doing. I went from thinking I would spend maybe a few hours with him every day to being afraid to leave him at home alone at all. This new revelation on this first day, this dawning that I needed to be with him much more than I had understood, was like driving down the road and the car shutting off suddenly. The resulting inertia caused whiplash. I was jerked forcefully into a new reality I had no idea how to deal with.

Over time I would learn more and settle into a somewhat structured routine, but it took a while.

On this first day, however, I was beginning to grasp just a bit of what I had signed up for when I agreed to be his caregiver because he adamantly refused to pay for one and didn't trust who the VA might send free of charge. In blunt terms, this meant that my caregiving services were free, and Dad could trust me. I learned during this season that while he did not have to pay for me caring for him, I had to pay for me caring for him. And the cost was starting to show just a bit on this first day.

I only got a tiny, fleeting preview, which was shocking because it was the first part of the process of my vision adjusting to see reality.

My phone conversation with the hospice company owner is how I discovered that I had faulty expectations about what was involved in the role of "caregiver" and what would be involved in the wide variety of decisions about his care facing me as he continued to decline. I was so naïve that I thought the caregiver role was limited to what a person with no medical knowledge could step into with nothing to offer but compassion and love for the patient. I literally assumed that what a caregiver did was provide companionship to the patient, be watchful to keep them safe, and perhaps do some cooking or cleaning and make sure the patient ate regularly. I truly believed that if a caregiver felt like their patient might need medical attention—assessment, intervention, or medication—they could contact the hospice company who would send a nurse to check and make sure they agreed with the caregiver's assessment and then coach the caregiver on giving whatever treatment was needed. I honestly thought this was how it would play out. I also thought the hospice nurse would keep me informed as to what to expect all along the way as the decline continued.

Instead, I discovered that as soon as I volunteered to be Dad's caregiver, I fully entered two different roles. Now I wasn't just the person solely responsible for all the details of his overall care. I was also the one giving the daily care as if he were a patient—my patient. Caregiving was <u>all</u> my responsibility, to bear alone.

This was a huge, heavy, awful, petrifying revelation.

I did decide to go home for the night late that evening because I knew I could not physically endure staying with him 24/7. I expected to spend about four hours with Dad, but I was with him for over nine hours on top of an additional hour to run errands for him. By the time I got home, my new reality was flexing its muscles. My journal entry at this time was so different from what I had typed up just that morning.

6/14/21 Late Night Journal Entry—

Why did I ever think I could do this? Who am I kidding?

I can't do this. Can't. Must.

Hours after I confidently predicted that all would be well because I knew God was with me, I began to understand that what I had taken on was going to be much more than I had envisioned. "Can't. Must." That was my new mantra adopted late in the evening of the first day of what would be a horrible, tumultuous, and scary time. A time of giving care, giving love, giving myself—all of myself. There simply was no other choice that was even remotely feasible to my heart. I had an overarching desire to do what was right to honor my dad, even when it meant the sacrifice of all I could possibly give.

I dug in deep for the duration, and I did the best I could.

But I had no idea what would be expected of me in the days, weeks, and months to come. I thought I knew it would be hard—I had no idea what hard was. I had absolutely no concept of the difficulty of the new reality that was to become my life. I had this naïve idea it would be a sweet time of bonding with him. Yes, there were some sweet moments that I cherish, but they were by far overshadowed by numerous times that held no sweetness.

I jumped into the hard and the ugly and the sharp edges and the isolation and the stress and the pressure and the dread and the hurt and the frustration and the looming unknowns that were always there.

I had heard friends' stories about the difficulty of caregiving for their parents. Back when I first realized that I would need to step up soon and make changes to accommodate Dad and keep him safe, I remember wondering what was wrong with me. I knew this was a common part of life—caring for aging parents—and others had done it and were doing it. *Why was I so stressed? Why was I terrified? Why was I already grieving the loss of my daddy?*

I was stressed because I was alone and, it turned out, completely uninformed. And this is important—when I say I was alone, I mean that literally. I'm single and an only child. My status added difficulty to an already difficult time. Also, I was faced with ever-increasing aging symptoms that I didn't know existed and surely didn't know how to handle. I was terrified because I was looking in the face of such an enormous responsibility to get this right, walking that fine line between taking charge and allowing him to think he was still in charge. After all, his autonomy and independence were vitally important to him, and he clung to any semblance of control tenaciously. And I was grieving because dementia was, bit by bit, stealing away the daddy I knew and replacing him with a very difficult-to-deal-with stranger.

I was carrying much more than I realized, and I just kept gradually adding to it. I didn't notice how heavy the load was becoming until I fell flat and started a cycle of falling over and over and having to continuously struggle to get back up with a load that kept getting heavier—again, and again, and again.

But by the grace of God, I kept scrambling and getting up, and I kept walking. I kept putting one foot in front of the other, taking a step or two, falling under the weight of what I carried, and getting up to take another step or two.

While I knew, logically, that this situation was temporary, only for a season, I got to a point where logic was lost at sea in the storm. And though it made no sense, nothing made sense anyway. I embraced a new belief system that I knew was flawed even as I believed it—this was not a season; this was forever.

This was not a season.
This was forever.

CHAPTER THREE

In Over My Head

Oh boy, was I ever in over my head here! My phone conversation with the hospice company owner on the first day of caregiving led to the startling realization of the vast distance between how I thought this would be and how it was turning out to be. That conversation triggered a landslide of all new emotions, fears, stress, and an intense feeling of being completely lost and overwhelmed.

When you are "green" about something, you have no experience with it, and you must learn. Then, there's being so green that you don't even know what questions to ask. To make things even harder, you discover that the little you thought you knew was useless and pretty much wrong. That was where I was, and there was no training manual, instruction book, or course to complete to emerge with a head full of new knowledge and a shiny bright certificate in my hand.

It was trial by fire—and my confidence had turned to ash.

I blindly moved toward a time of helping my dad along the path to the end of his life. I didn't realize I had no sight until it became obvious that my perception held only vague shadows, indistinguishable shapes, and inky blackness. Yet, in my blindness, I was expected to navigate an impossible path to an unknown destination filled with numerous unknown stops along the way. I know that sounds dramatic, but that is how it felt to me. I had no guidance or details of what to expect. Just darkness.

I tried a couple of strategies to push the darkness back. I did online research but could not find what I was looking for. Yes, I came across all sorts of advice, but none about a situation similar to what I faced with my dad. Though he was caught in the throes of dementia, he was still very alert and aware. He was also hyper-vigilantly watchful for anything that appeared to him to be a situation where he was purposely not being included when he should be.

Dad insisted on being completely involved in every detail of his care, which was fine, except when it came to things he thought he understood that he did not. In addition to online research, I talked to people who had dealt with aging loved ones, but none were or had been in a situation that mirrored mine. I learned quickly that the two roles I took on—caregiving and care decision-making—overlapped. I had to be two people at once and often acted simultaneously as his only caregiver and only care decision-maker. I've always been fairly proficient at multi-tasking.

But this? This was a whole new level, and I kept running into walls, wiping out around curves, and flying out into an unknown black hole that seemed to swallow me on repeat.

Let's back up a bit and retrace our steps down the path that led to that fateful conversation with the hospice company owner on my first day of caregiving.

In late 2020, I had several conversations with my dad's doctor, who I thought would be a source of support and encouragement while offering insights from his many years of experience with aging patients. Unfortunately, that didn't happen at anywhere near the level that I longed for. In hindsight, I'm not sure why I expected more support from him. I think I was reaching out for support wherever I thought I might receive it because I felt so alone in this and was desperate for help.

After a hospital stay in early June of 2021, Dad's doctor wanted to see him, and surprisingly, he allowed me to take him. He had canceled previous doctor's appointments and had chosen to discontinue all his medications, so I was shocked when he agreed to go. It was at this doctor's visit

This was a whole new level, and I kept running into walls, wiping out around curves, and flying out into an unknown black hole that seemed to swallow me on repeat.

that the doctor took me aside and recommended another way for Dad to be cared for. He started this conversation by giving me a brutal scenario: "Your dad could have a heart attack and fall. When EMS comes, they would run in, break his ribs, shock his heart, and then rush him to the hospital, where he would be placed on a ventilator, and he may or may not recover. This scenario happens too often with age, and it can be avoided by opting for him to be cared for by home hospice instead."

I had no words to answer him with. It was as if he had thrown ice-cold water on me. This picture he painted was shocking.

He recommended a particular company and said they would send nurses to check his vitals twice a week. He added, "This strategy will allow your dad to stay in his home where he is most comfortable instead of being repeatedly in and out of the hospital. Your father's Medicare insurance will pay for this service."

"Okay," I agreed, "I guess this next step makes sense." We chatted a moment more, then told my dad together.

The doctor presented the idea to Dad by starting with the same heart attack scenario, which only confused him. The doctor attempted to clarify with something Dad was familiar with: "The Afib issue you have had intermittently for years could result in a stroke or a heart attack at some point.

The medications from your cardiologist to stop the erratic heartbeat may not always work."

"Are you saying I have a bad heart?" my dad asked him, still confused.

"Yes, Mr. Lund. You have a bad heart," he answered matter-of-factly.

Looking back, I feel sure the doctor used this absolute worst-case scenario strategy for the shock value to ensure we (mainly Dad) would be open to starting home hospice. I don't believe this was helpful at all to that end. While Dad did have Afib episodes, I don't agree that he necessarily had a bad heart. The doctor's choice to present this care alternative in this way only added to my father's ongoing stress, mistrust, and confusion. But once we both understood the general idea of how home hospice services would work, we told the doctor we would discuss this further, make a decision, and I would let him know the result.

Regardless of how it was presented, this hospice care solution sounded so simple. It felt like an answer. The rest of Dad's resistance faded when he learned that Medicare paid for this service. We discussed it later in the evening, and Dad agreed to allow me to set it up.

I felt hopeful.

I truly believed that it would be helpful for Dad—and helpful for me too.

But home hospice services were not at all simple or helpful. Why? Because I didn't know what I didn't know. I think I was probably more clueless than the average person, but I will lay it all out and reveal just how little I understood because there may be someone else out there like me.

Here's what I knew:

- I knew hospice care had a couple of levels. I knew that someone with a terminal illness received hospice care after all medical alternatives had been exhausted.

- I knew hospice nurses made the patient as comfortable as possible until they passed away.

- I knew that "in-home hospice care" was a level of care that could be provided when a patient was declining but before death was imminent.

- I also knew that when in-home hospice services began, a "care package" was kept in the home for the patient. This was a bag of prescription medications commonly used by in-home hospice patients in varying stages of decline.

Here is what I did not know:

- I did not know what was included with this level of hospice service and what was not.

- I did not know what hospice nurses
  providing this care did and did not do.

- I did not know what the hospice
  doctor did and did not do.

- I also did not know how a caregiver fit
  in with in-home hospice services.

The logistics of caregiver services were a key concept I did not understand. I did not realize that while Medicare paid for the basic in-home hospice services, they did not pay any part of the cost for a caregiver to stay with the patient. So not only did I not have any understanding of what the caregiver role entailed, but I also did not realize that Medicare did not help with any costs if it was determined that a caregiver was needed.

Bottom line—I had some puzzle pieces here, but I had no idea how they all fit together. I knew hospice nurses checked on their patients. I knew medications were kept on hand in the home in case they were needed. I knew that caregivers stayed in the home with the patient if they could not be safe alone. That's where my knowledge stopped, and unfortunately, I allowed assumptions to fill in the gaps.

- I *assumed* that hospice nurses did everything
  nurses do, including determining when
  to give care package medications after
  checking out the patient in person.

- I *assumed* that a hospice physician or the patient's regular doctor would be available for face-to-face visits if the patient could leave home to go to a doctor's office while under hospice care.

- I *assumed* hospice personnel would provide ongoing help and support for me as Dad's caregiver and care decision-maker by offering knowledge gained from their education and experience working with aging patients.

Because I lacked so much understanding, I looked forward to starting at-home hospice service. I anticipated relief from the stress that had been gradually increasing for a long time with Dad as I saw more and more that he was declining.

Right after the hospice company's initial assessment, and a couple of days before I started officially being Dad's caregiver, I wrote this in my journal:

6/12/21 Journal Entry—

I thought hospice care would be like a nice, warm blanket on a bitterly cold day. Comforting. Helpful. Beneficial. Peaceful. Nope. It's all sharp edges and new uncharted territory and overwhelming information and people who, to be honest, so far I'm not very impressed with ... yet. I do believe they are trying. But they don't know Dad, and they don't know me.

My assumptions and expectations were entirely faulty and unrealistic. I think I knew this immediately at some level, but I had no idea how much I didn't know at first. I had these fantasies in my head of how this was going to be that just weren't true. I thought this hospice company would come in and take over and make informed recommendations and suggestions for every step of this process. I thought interacting with them would look something like this:

- They were health care professionals looking after a patient.

- I was like a visitor in the hospital, keeping the patient company and tending to non-medical needs to lend support. I did not feel at all qualified to administer treatment or make medical decisions.

- I knew I might have to make that call sometimes, but I expected informed recommendations and specific instructions.

But I soon learned just how far away I was from reality.

Unfortunately, the hospice company that my dad's doctor recommended turned out not to be a good fit, which complicated things even more. After a month, I changed companies, which meant starting all over again with an assessment and getting to know new people and their way of doing things. I should have made the switch much sooner, but because I was so new at all of this, I initially thought the problem was me. I second-guessed the miscommunication, confusion, and frustration I felt, attributing it to my lack of experience. Also, Dad was so very averse to any type of change in his routine by this time that my desire to keep limping along with this same company increased. I kept thinking it would get better, and instead, it kept getting worse. I did talk to Dad a couple of times about my concerns, and he made it clear he thought I was overreacting.

Of course, I never told Dad all the details. For example, I got a phone call from the hospice company's chaplain soon after hospice care began. He informed me that he was on his way to Dad's and would arrive in a few minutes.

"I'm sorry, sir, but that won't work," I said, " Dad is taking a nap, so now is not a good time."

"Ma'am, there is just a five-day 'grace period' for chaplain services. I am already in the area and on my way to your dad's home. I'll be there shortly."

"Sir, I need you to choose another day," I insisted, "Dad needs his rest, and he can't go back to sleep when a nap is interrupted." Then the conversation escalated to the point that I don't remember what all he said, but I do remember pointing out to him that he was a chaplain, and he was being harsh with me.

"Well, you are being harsh and unprofessional with me," he responded.

Wow. I was the brand new caregiver who was already over-stressed, and my stress was showing. He was a chaplain who should have been a calming and comforting presence, and instead, he was demanding, rude, and impatient. So there was that.

Another example of their less-than-acceptable level of service was their miscommunication about a male nurse for Dad. I had made it abundantly clear to the owner at the very beginning that Dad refused even to consider having a male nurse. It didn't matter whether or not this was a rational request. He was sick and old, and this was his preference. She had assured me that this would be no problem. But one day, when the assigned nurse was unavailable, a male nurse showed up, and I had to explain why I could not allow him to come in and then ask him to leave. He was very nice about it. But his time was wasted driving over, which should not have happened. I called, and the owner did apologize, but she blamed "the office" for the miscommunication. And then, she told me, "The company office is actually pretty far away from you." She added, "We are located on the other side of Houston. There are only two nurses who live near your area, and one of them is a man."

I was shocked at this. "Wow. This is concerning," I said. "Why didn't you tell me this might be a problem when I first told you my father is uncomfortable with male nurses? You said that was not an issue, and I took you at your word."

She explained, "We have plenty of other female nurses. If the female nurse in your area is unavailable, you will just have to wait an hour or so for one to arrive."

This was even more concerning to me. "What if it is an emergency situation?" I asked.

She calmly replied, "Oh, the nurse will instruct you on what to do in an emergency." As if that would make me feel better.

No, it only added to the weight on my shoulders that kept getting heavier.

I could go on with examples, but you get the point. Typing this all out now, I can't believe I did not immediately switch companies, but I trust myself a lot more now than I did then.

Caregiving is a nuanced role. There were many complexities in dealing with my dad. For example, his ongoing concern about being left out of any detail of his care. These suspicions grew when hospice nurses began coming by. When the nurse addressed me, I always had to be careful to keep directing her back to speak with him. Add to this dilemma that Dad would not wear his hearing aids, and the result was a difficult hurdle to jump over every time a nurse came by. If the nurse spoke too loudly, he would accuse her of yelling at him. Too softly, and he could not hear her. I could not even walk the nurse to the door as she left because that aroused Dad's suspicions that we were having a private conversation and leaving him out. I also learned quickly that it was best for me not to talk on the phone at all unless it was absolutely necessary, because even if he was sleeping, sometimes he would wake up, and he always wanted to know who I was talking to and what I might be not including him in. While I empathize with how difficult it must be to lose your autonomy, his lack of trust in me to act in his best interests and on his behalf added to the daily stress of my new life.

> Dad's lack of trust in me to act in his best interests and on his behalf added to the daily stress of my new life.

Dad was also very focused on his financial status, a practice he had honed for years. He closely monitored his finances and wanted to see all his bank statements and investment company statements. This was not a bad thing, but because he was used to being completely in control of how his money was spent, he did not permit me to use his funds to pay for any of his needs now like I had heard that several of my friends and family had done for their aging parents. They would hire caregivers and just take the payments out of the account in the name of the parent they were overseeing care for, and their parent did not object or even question them at all. This was not an option for me. Instead, I was limited to lying to him about how much something cost and paying the difference myself or telling him the truth, knowing he would not allow me to use his funds. I chose honesty for most things, including caregiving expenses.

A week after this hospice service started, Dad suddenly got extremely congested. He had been fine all day long. He was fine when I left him for the night and went home, but he called me just a few minutes after I got home. He sounded croupy. He was wheezing and struggling to breathe, which made him anxious. I rushed back to his house and did what I was supposed to do—call the hospice company.

The nurse who lived in the area was unavailable, and the ETA for another nurse was at least an hour, possibly longer. Dad was laboring to breathe and panicking, and I was too. I had never heard him like this before. So, I canceled the hospice nurse and took him to the Emergency Room. They admitted him, and he stayed in the hospital for a few days. When his doctor came by on rounds, I learned more hard truths about in-home hospice services and more of what was expected of me as Dad's care decision-maker and caregiver.

CHAPTER FOUR

Nurse in Training With No Training

Canceling the hospice nurse was difficult, but I was confident I had made the right decision. I felt relieved when they took him straight back, got him on oxygen, and started trying to determine what was going on. But according to Dad's doctor, I made the wrong decision. When he came by and spoke with us on his hospital rounds a day or two later, he made it very clear that I could have waited for the hospice nurse to arrive. He went so far as to strongly imply that I should have waited—saying it without directly stating it.

Wait ... what???

"The morphine in the care package would have been helpful had you given him a dose," he said. "Morphine is not only for pain, but it can also be used for anxiety. A dose of morphine would have calmed him down, which would have also helped his breathing issues while waiting for the hospice nurse to arrive."

"I didn't know that," I said.

He seemed incredulous that I didn't know, as if he was thinking, *"How could she not have known this?"* And then he made this statement: "Staying out of the hospital is one of the main goals of in-home hospice care," I nodded my head, feeling like a scolded child or a less-than-intelligent human being. *I get that,* I thought, *but sorry, if my daddy is struggling to breathe, he's not the only one dealing with anxiety over this. I was freaking out too!* Of course, it didn't help that I didn't pay attention when the hospice nurse very quickly went over all the care package medications because, in my clueless dream world, I thought <u>she</u> would be the one to give the first dose of each of them and then give me hands-on training for future doses. I was not told that I would be responsible for administering all care package medications. Maybe the nurse thought I knew. Perhaps other people have this knowledge, but I definitely did not. And if she said that morphine could be for anxiety, too, I missed that completely. I missed a whole lot completely.

> I missed a whole lot completely.

When the doctor told me all this, I began to see more of my new reality. And it scared me to death.

I will never know if being with a different hospice company from the beginning might have resulted in a better grasp of how the medications worked and what my responsibilities were for administering them, but this is how it played out for us.

When the doctor crashed through my fantasy world with this terrifying new reality, this is what I learned: a caregiver is an entry-level nurse with no training at all unless they happen to work in the medical field or for a caregiver company or make a living as a caregiver on their own. Having never been exposed to caregiving, I went in with absolutely no foundation for this, no point of reference, no comparison point. I was to be a confident, brave soul with no expertise in what I had volunteered to do and no perception of what my daily life would be like. Sure, I could call and talk to someone from the hospice company if I had questions, but I was alone dealing with their answers and deciding whether or not they would work for my dad. As Dad's caregiver, I was the one expected to administer care package medications when needed. I was the one to encourage him to try Thick-It to help him with swallowing issues that he denied he had. I was the one who had to try various ways suggested to help him swallow pills (if he even agreed to take them). I was the one … for everything.

And as the sole decision maker for his care, I also had to decide how long it was safe to leave him alone while attempting to take care of myself.

No one had prepared me for how hard this was going to be. Or how lonely.

I learned the hard way that a caregiver who is an immediate family member is usually the one who gets all the pushback from the patient. Their fear. Their anger. Their frustration. It all needed release, and here was the easy target. Yep. That would be me.

Dad had no understanding of what his status was. He thought (adamantly) that he was fine staying alone and refused to allow anyone else to be with him other than, of course, me. I know others have been in this situation and forced the issue, but I chose not to do that. Looking back, though my decision made it almost impossibly hard for me, it was the right decision for us. I know without a doubt that Dad would have made everything worse for me and himself if I had tried to force the issue of allowing others to stay with him. That said, it's true that someone else helping out would have given me a much-needed reprieve. On my own, my only "break" was occasionally running around the corner to my home briefly while he took a nap, and if he was doing okay throughout the day, I tried sleeping at least a few hours at night in my own bed. But this reprieve I could have received would have come at a great cost. Had I entrusted Dad's care to anyone else, my time with him would have been even more stressful and tension-filled. The cost was too high.

Another problem with Dad's mindset was that he believed that he would get better. He thought he had an illness that he would recover fully from. He asked me several times throughout this caregiving season how long I was going to continue taking care of him. As weeks turned into months, Dad kept asking, "When am I going to get better?"

It was heartbreaking.

6/16/21 Journal Entry—

I figured out today that Dad thinks that all of this current arrangement, including my caregiving, is temporary. He's asked me several times this week since the hospice company did the initial assessment on 6/11 how long I'll be doing this, and I just say, "As long as it takes." He thinks all of this arrangement is related to AFib (irregular heartbeat that he was in the hospital for right before hospice services started) and believes if he does not have AFib again for however long, hospice will end. He keeps telling me I'm giving up my life and says I can't keep doing it, yet when I mention that people have offered to come by and be with him when I need to go somewhere, he says he's fine alone and doesn't need a babysitter.

He said tonight that if he doesn't have AFib again, he can get back to what he was doing, staying alone, and I can go back to my life. Ummm … no. Not happening. But I cannot tell him.

What could I say? I could not tell him that this arrangement would last until he died. He sometimes knew he was dying, but many times he did not understand this, not until very close to the end. When he would also ask me why he wasn't getting better or adamantly insist that he had to go to his doctor or the ER so that he could get better, I would just say, "Dad, only God knows when you will get better." We were already doing everything that would be done for him by a doctor or medical staff in the hospital.

He grew increasingly stubborn about medication. He periodically needed medication for his congestion, cough, and digestive issues, but he mostly refused to take it. He had a lifelong problem with swallowing pills that only intensified during this season, and liquid medications were not an option either because, according to him, they burned his throat "like fire." Occasionally he could get a pill down successfully, but for the most part, he would either gag and spit it out, or it would get stuck in his throat. Crushing pills didn't work because no matter what I put it in (and I tried *everything* suggested and more), he insisted he could taste it and would refuse it. When a pill got stuck, Dad would complain about that and the bitter taste lingering. He made sure he reported to me periodically that the bad taste was still there. He would keep complaining about whatever the medication did to him for hours, saying, "I want you to understand how horrible this is!"

Each time a medication dose didn't go well, Dad would insist he would not take any more. Understandably, every time he had an issue requiring any medication, it served as a trigger for me, greatly increasing my ongoing, daily dread.

I knew going in that this would not be easy. I could not know the level of impossible that would be reached so quickly and continue rising each day. I can look back now, read my journal entries, and marvel at how God pulled me through this. Otherwise, there was no way I would have made it through and been able to honor Dad's wish to be his only caregiver and let him leave this earth from his home.

I knew this would not be easy—I could not know the level of impossible it would become ...

ENCOURAGEMENT FROM THE LORD

"From the end of the earth
I will cry to You,
When my heart is overwhelmed;
Lead me to the rock that is higher than I."

PSALM 61:2, NKJV

CHAPTER FIVE

This is Hell

ONE WEEK AFTER BECOMING DAD'S CAREGIVER

6/21/21 Journal Entry—

This is hell. No, wait, that was nothing. <u>This</u> is hell. No, wait, all that was a walk in the park. **This** is hell. No, wait, <u>**THIS**</u> is hell. No, wait …

One week down, fifteen more weeks to go (though I didn't know that then), and already I was thinking like this. Overdramatic? Sure, but also intensely real. This is how I felt, all the way down deep—and this quickly. The evening before had been horrible. Dad and I had a conversation that turned into a heated and lengthy "discussion."

Unfortunately, this was only my first experience like this, with many more to come.

This time gave me my first lesson on how quickly and adamantly Dad could totally change his mind. During his most recent hospital stay which was right after hospice services began, we talked about getting a caregiver for the night shift after he came home. When we discussed this in his hospital room, he seemed surprisingly open to letting me investigate further. He was even amiable about it while in the hospital. But that all changed drastically the evening I got him home. I planned to stay that night with him and then try to get a caregiver set up soon after. But I discovered his mindset had changed, creating a late-evening, frustrating encounter.

6/21/21 Journal Entry (Continued)—

Last night, I got him home and settled, and then I went home for a bit before coming back to spend the night. I called a caregiver that a cousin had given me contact information for and talked to her. She was very nice and quoted me pricing that was about half the going hourly rate. After I got my stuff done at home, I went back over to Dad's around 8:30 p.m. Around 9:00, I broached the subject of getting a caregiver set up for the night shift like we had discussed in the hospital, and I told him about the caregiver I had talked to when I went home. He knew her from when she cared for my aunt, and he liked her. It seemed like a great solution.

Ha.

Because I knew he would ask, I went ahead and told him honestly how much she charged and explained that it was significantly less than the going rate.

And then, we "talked" for two hours. In circles. With escalating emotion. His attitude about this had completely changed. COMPLETELY. He refused to get a caregiver for the night shift, period. And he even refused to do the Medic Alert system we had talked about before that he had been agreeable to. We had been together in the hospital, with little sleep, for two nights. We were exhausted and arguing and kept being exhausted and arguing. And it got very heated, over and over. Round and round with no way out. On and on and on … and on … We didn't really resolve anything, but we finally gave up and let exhaustion take over, and he went to bed. I got ready for a long night on the couch.

Unfortunately, the next morning was no better. We stayed strained and tense all morning. No matter what I did, it was wrong. The night before, we finally went to bed around 11:00 p.m., and I got up early in the morning, went home to shower, and came back. When I returned, I was in a hurry because the hospice nurse was supposed to be there soon, and I wanted to be sure Dad was up and fully awake and had plenty of time to have breakfast before she came. Silly me. I rushed inside without realizing it, and he immediately picked up on that. "What are you rushing around like that for?" He said in a sharp tone.

"I'm sorry, Dad, I didn't realize I was rushing," I said.

"Well, I guess we are starting out again, just like last night," he replied.

"No, Dad, we aren't," I responded, "I won't allow it. *'This is the day that the Lord has made; let us rejoice and be glad in it.'*[1] Let's choose to have a better outlook today. We have a lot to be grateful for."

But my attempt to bring about a fresh perspective failed, and our morning flew downhill from there. There was no changing his choice to complain and criticize. By the time I began fixing his breakfast in the kitchen, I was fighting tears and talking in my head about being in hell.

And then, I made another significant mistake. I presented an option I thought would be very helpful and lift his sour mood, but my timing was all wrong. During the long sleepless night on his couch, I replayed our "discussion" and got to the part where I had told him that if he refused another caregiver for the night shift, I would have to stay with him at night as well as during the day. I hoped he would realize how serious I was about him not being alone at night and give in. Why would I think that? I should have known better. And during that exhausting late night/early morning on his lumpy couch, I fully realized the impossibility of that option. Who was I kidding? I could not physically do that, not to mention emotionally handle how draining it would be. So I decided to back off on trying to get him set up with a caregiver at night as long as he would agree to allow me to set up a Medic Alert system.

I realize now that choosing to tell him my new revelation the next morning was a terrible idea because the air between us was still tense after a tough night. I truly believed this was something he would want to hear and appreciate, and I hoped this new idea I was suggesting would alleviate the palpable tension between us and, therefore, lessen the strain of the day. I thought this was a great compromise that would help us meet in the middle.

It didn't work out that way at all. Dad accused me of not wanting to be around him, and he said he felt like I could not wait to escape him. *What???* And this launched another heated discussion, already.

The rest of that day was varying degrees of strong verbal volleying back and forth with a few breaks. The breaks were forced upon us because we were both too weary to keep going without backing off a little bit here and there. By that night when I left to go home to bed for a few hours, he thought I would not be back the next day, or ever, even though I had not said anything to that effect. He was super touchy, confused, frustrated, and exhausted. I wasn't much better.

It felt like hell.

This scenario of being unable to do or say *anything* right would repeat itself frequently. This day was just another one of many times.

I will say that with lots of prayer and practice, I got somewhat better at handling this recurring challenge. I learned some new strategies for responding to his no-holds-barred emotional outbursts, complete with sarcasm, full-on negativity, and dissatisfaction with my efforts. But for every one or two times I reacted in a healthier way, I also tended to run backward and get drawn into this insane circular race just as much, if not more, the next time. It was so hard not to allow his harsh words to elicit an emotional response. He was the one with personality-altering dementia, but I found myself acting like I was insane. Because in those moments, I was.

I would often respond with kind words, but he quickly picked up on my tone and/or expression and accused me of being angry. Busted. But I would not admit it because that only made things worse. If I did not reply at all, that fed his anger too. Even the most healthy, kind, and calm reaction to one of his tirades could backfire intensely. A reply that might work well one time exploded in my face the next time. I never knew what to expect because his actions and reactions were not predictable—at all—ever. That common-sense strategy of trying to learn something from a previous experience so that you don't repeat what didn't work? That was useless in this season. I just had to do my best, even though my best was usually not good enough. My best was all I had.

By that night, I felt so defeated and discouraged, and my journal entry reflected that.

6/21/21 Journal Entry (continued)—

I don't want to talk to anyone. I want to isolate. I want to numb out. I want to disappear. But I have to give care. And I have to provide care to the touchiest person on the face of the earth. And I don't know what I'm doing. But that does not matter. I have to learn. Lord, I know that I'm breaking down, and maybe that's a good thing because then, to stand, I will have to lean on You.

6/22/21 Journal Entry (the next morning)—

I'm done with telling myself I just need to suck it up and do what I have to do. That's useless. I have to get to the place where I start trusting and relying on God instead of doing it on my own.

I knew the right answers. I knew what needed to happen. Adversity should bring about more reliance on God. More reliance on God should bring sorely needed rest to my soul. But I was already beginning to see that for me it wasn't working out that way. Oh, how I longed to rest in and fully trust Him. I was so worn out so quickly, and there was no end in sight. There was also no magic button I could push to make what I so deeply desired a reality in my life. It was hard work, seeking God and carrying an unquenched thirst for His presence and reassurance. I was so thirsty. Despite all my efforts and heartfelt prayers, I never experienced a supernatural shift to a consistently positive and hopeful outlook. I did choose to hold tight to any glimmer of light that came, no matter how small, but any reprieve was fleeting.

This completely different way of moving through each day was all there was. Life before seemed like a distant memory. I trudged on. Two excruciating months went by, and after a particularly tough day, I went to my journal.

8/22/21 Journal Entry—

This is hell. Or, just more intensity of complete awfulness. Totally complete awfulness until there seems to be no room for more, but more will come.

About two weeks later, at close to three months in, I was deep into the oppressing darkness. And by now, I really could not leave Dad, hardly at all.

9/5/21 Journal Entry—

This is what depression looks and feels like. Dread so heavy it's crushing. Sleep that is not restful, relaxing, or enjoyable, and awakening slowly, like I've been drugged. Stress is so overpowering and continual, with no end. My focus every day is just to get through it. At the same time, I have to work on things and figure stuff out I have no clue about and make decisions that are so hard and huge and menacing and scary. I don't know if I can keep going like this, but it just adds more pressure to continue to consider other options that don't look promising or in any way helpful to all I'm dealing with. I have nothing left.

It occurs to me that throughout all these weeks, I had choices not to be so completely isolated. I could have arranged to meet with friends during a regular break in the day when he was taking a nap. I could have probably gone to church or small group, at least occasionally. But I found it too stressful and exhausting even to consider these options. It's easier to stay in familiar hell than to try to break out here and there because there really is no break where you are free of it, and you always must go back into the midst of it. I stayed all in completely isolated, thinking that was best.

It might have been best. But now it's all I have. It's all I am.

9/8/21 Journal Entry—

So tired I literally can hardly move. I just may not survive today. It's one of those really overwhelming exhaustion and stress and tears behind my eyelids days. Lovely. God, I want to cry so badly. I'm just that tired and stressed and overwhelmed today. But crying is useless, a waste of time, and I have no time anyway.

More deep darkness went by, and by mid-September, I felt hopeless.

9/14/21 Journal Entry—

THIS, NOT ANYTHING BEFORE THIS, IS MY ENTRANCE INTO HELL. Everything preceding this was a walk in the park.

Three days later.

9/17/21 Journal Entry—

I feel like I'm in a forever form of some level of hell.

I'm an epic failure at all of this. I hate it. I love him, but it's just too foreign and just … hard. And it's not me. Definitely not my natural bent.

Today, just like every day, all my responses, every angle I tried, failed. Made no difference. At all.

I've decided that this is a very basic first level of hell to make me more thankful for where I will be in eternity.

> "This is hell" was hell.

"This is hell" was hell. The worst of the worst kept somehow impossibly getting worse. And worse.

And worse.

I didn't think it could get worse than … and then it would. It was like I kept falling down, and the injury kept getting re-wounded again, more and more. The wounds were deeper and more painful. My emotions kept coming up, surfacing all over and around and under and deep within, more and more, until I stopped being shocked and stricken. I resigned myself to living in an earthly level of hell. And I resigned myself to living there indefinitely. I just existed. Ash heaps remain in the fallout, and they can still smolder when I bring these days to mind.

Maybe they always will.

I had never been a negative person, but these were my raw, unfiltered, very real reactions during this season. Was it right? Was it how I was supposed to react in a tough situation, especially when I factor in that I am a committed Christian?

Initially, I felt guilty. The intense pressure I lived with brought out some ugly realizations. Who I thought I was as a Christian, where I thought I stood at this point in my life, and how I always envisioned I would act and react when life got hard was completely different from my shocking and disappointing reality.

But God.

ENDNOTE

1   Psalm 118:24.

ENCOURAGEMENT FROM THE LORD

*"He lifted me out of the pit of despair,
out of the mud and the mire.*

*He set my feet on solid ground and
steadied me as I walked along.*

PSALM 40:2, NLT

CHAPTER SIX

Awful

7/8/21 Journal Entry—

Every single day is awful at some level. Even better days have something awful in them. I want to embrace this season. Move through it obediently. I am being obedient to what I feel that God has called me to do.

But I can't embrace awful. I'm trying. It's not happening.

Instead, I dread it, and hate it, and long for its end. But the only end is just a new kind of awful. Death. Grief. I should not want the end. That's wrong.

I'm so tired of awful. But it's all there is. And it will continue indefinitely.

No matter how hard I tried, I could not embrace awful. It was prickly and sharp, and it adamantly did not want to be hugged. It wanted to be awful.

> There truly was some awful in every single day.

Within a few short weeks, I learned a lot about my new way of living. I learned that there were no good days. Good moments? Yes. But entire days that were good? No. What I learned was: There were really bad days, bad days, and better days. There truly was some awful in every single day.

I lived just two streets over from Dad. Soon after becoming his caregiver, I set up a Medic Alert system for him. For these reasons, I was so fortunate that, for the most part during this season, I had the opportunity to sleep in my own bed at home at night for at least a few hours. Sleeping in my own bed—even for a short time—was helpful. It provided a mental separation from my dad, and I needed that desperately. Yet any time spent at home away from him typically included heavy dread. I dreaded a new time of awful when I returned to him. As I headed back to his house, I wondered what would greet me when I opened his door. Anger? Depression? Frustration? Confusion? Or maybe a smile and kindness, at least briefly. I just never knew. So I dreaded opening that door to find out.

This dread started months before I became his caregiver, when I was still working full-time but regularly going by his home to check on him. His house was dark and dirty and felt oppressive. On the weekends, I tended to put off going over there as long as possible and then felt bad for doing that. I didn't want to enter his world. Selfish. But real. Let me share with you an excerpt from my journal during this time:

5/1/21 (Saturday) Journal Entry—

It's almost 3:00 p.m., and I haven't called Dad yet ... because I don't want to go over there and enter into his life and feel all the bad stuff. Super duper selfish. I'm honest, so I'll admit that I do this every time—do my thing and then dread calling him and going over there. But at some point, I take a deep breath, and I make that call.

Even before I began caregiving full-time, spending time in his home felt much like spending time in a dungeon. Even if he was in a good mood, the state of his home made me feel like the walls were closing in.

Once I was there as his caregiver for most of every day, I realized that there was no logical way to prepare myself for how the day might go, because dementia has no logic. There was no briefing. I had no idea if today would have some good mood vibes and maybe a few treasured sweet moments or not. And if not, I had to dig deep to do my best not to react in anger or tears or shut down because if I did any of these things, it made an extremely difficult situation worse. He would react to my reaction and start a vicious cycle of us reacting to each other repeatedly.

Awful.

I so wanted to do what I have done for many years when faced with a tough situation—grit my teeth and push through it. Tough it out and get to the other side. Keep pushing myself hard. But I found that there was no push left within me after just a short time. A very short time. I was depleted so quickly, and that discouraged me. All that was left was the get through it part, whatever that looked like, and it looked struggle-filled at some level every day.

Every. Day.

A wonderful girlfriend gave me a little book called *Prayers of Hope for Caregivers*. It had daily encouragement and prayers for a wide variety of caregiving situations. Some did not apply to me, but the ones that did really did. One of the entries referred to feeling as though you are trapped. In captivity.[1] Yes. That's exactly how I felt. A captive, staying in a dungeon for hours every day, trying to help my dad while also trying to remain calm and kind and safely detached regardless of what I faced. I failed. Over and over and over. But regardless of what happened each day, I had to start again the next day with no idea what challenges I would encounter.

Awful.

6/26/21 Journal Entry—

It's so sad when you sleep well but wake up feeling like you're going to throw up because you have to face another day. When you're having some tingling pre-panic symptoms for no reason except you just don't want to be here forcing yourself to do this. Tears on the edge—threatening to spill over, but they can't because there's no time for that, and I feel like it's whining that is useless anyway.

I don't feel like this every morning, thank God, but it's here big and ugly today. Exhaustion and dread and sadness and heaviness weighing down hard. Nothing different has happened. I just don't want to do my new day-in-day-out-same-thing. Don't want to do any of the daily stuff for Dad I've committed to do. But this is my life.

I do want to honor Dad. I do want to do this right thing. I do. But it's too much. It's overwhelming. I feel like I'm lying flat in the dust, being run over, over and over again, all day long, every day.

Lord, I need You.

7/6/21 Journal Entry—

I usually sleep pretty good, but I feel like I don't. And when I have been sleeping, and I wake up, there are a few moments of normal, followed by the realization of my life now. That gut punch feeling of … oh, yeah, this is where I am. This must be my new normal for an indefinite, maybe very long indefinite, period of time. And then I begin the countdown of how long I have until I have to get up and face another day of this new normal. And the dread builds.

8/3/21 Journal Entry—

Rough night. Hard time going to sleep to begin with. Instead, I went there, to the hard places, and allowed the crushing weight of everything to feel as crushing as it is. I try not to dwell on it, to fret or whatever over it, just try to keep going and do the next thing. But sometimes, like last night, I go there all the way. I was just lying there wide awake. Not so much running scenarios in my head like I usually do, not last night. Just feeling the weight all the way. Heavy and cumbersome and stressful and pressure-filled and dreadful.

Dread is always present. Mainly every morning. Mornings are hard. Knowing that I must discipline myself to embark on another day of awful. Lying in bed each morning knowing I will need to get up soon and get ready and put on my caregiver role uniform and take ownership of what's heavy upon me. Again. Every day.

The responsibility is always there, of course, whether I'm physically with Dad or not. But when I'm there at Dad's, it's front and center and everywhere.

The weight of the weight. The wait of the wait. The wait of the weight. And the weight of the wait.

⁂

The weight of the weight.

The wait of the wait.

The wait of the weight.

And the weight of the wait.

⁂

Awful.

I thought it might be helpful to others in this situation to include a little synopsis here—just a general idea of what daily life with my dad was like. A look into my daily awful. I think it might have helped me had I known others had similar experiences and felt the same way that I did. It might have eased the burden of doubt, of dread, even of guilt for my doubt and my dread.

Dad was always picky—a perfectionist. But now I couldn't do his toast right. And I had too much jam on his toast, or not enough. And the blasted toaster oven was how to toast everything. Because it tasted better toasted in there when it was done right. But I so rarely did it right.

As crazy as it sounds, after Dad passed away, I made a little ceremony out of throwing that despicable toaster oven away when I cleaned out his house. It was a symbol of my misery, and now I was taking back control. It felt so good to throw it in the trash.

I couldn't even boil the water with the tea bags and mix up his tea to his satisfaction consistently, even though I was extra careful to do it the same way each time.

Almost every time I cooked for him, something wasn't as it should be. He would usually eat but complain about whatever he saw as the problem with the food, and I knew that meant there was no point in freezing it for leftovers. Really, even if what I cooked didn't turn out perfect, it was okay, or at the very least, edible. I'll be the first to say I'm not a good cook, but nothing I set before him was so bad that it deserved that level of complaint.

In fact, that I cooked for him should have sparked gratitude and an appreciative willingness to overlook what wasn't perfect.

It should have, but it didn't.

He was anxious before. Looking back, I learned that anxiety was almost always underneath his anger. Grabbing onto power and control to cover up the fear. But now, now he was terrified. He was anxious about being dropped when he was assisted in getting up. He would say, "You're going to drop me!" often. He said this to me but also to medical personnel, which gave me some level of comfort that I wasn't assisting him incorrectly. He was also afraid of running out of money, which was an invalid concern. Because of this fear, we often had to go over how much money he had in the bank and in his investments. And because of his dementia, we couldn't go over it just once; we had to do it repeatedly because he had trouble understanding how much he had where. In general, it was obvious that he was afraid of losing control of his life, and his control was slipping away more and more at a rapid rate. Now, his anxiety was still cloaked in anger, but because there was so much more fear, there was a lot more anger to cover it up when he could. So that meant more intense frustration proclamations and explosive angry outbursts.

He had ongoing issues with the temperature in the house. He was too cold or too warm all day long, every single day. He adamantly insisted that I use his AC and heat to regulate what was not possible to regulate. He had no comprehension that running the heat in the mornings during the summer to "get the chill out" does not make sense. When he could no longer adjust the temperature himself, I learned quickly to turn the heat on as soon as I arrived in the morning. Right after we said good morning, he would ask me if I had turned the heat on, and he would be incredulous and upset with me if I hadn't because … "Can't you tell it's cold in this house?"

So, I would run the heat for a little while every day and suffer. A few minutes or sometimes a few hours later, he would be too warm and want a fan running and the AC on and turned down. Then he would get cold and want a blanket and socks, and he wanted me to turn the fan off and the AC temperature up. Then he would get too hot again. We went through numerous cycles of this every day. He also asked me repeatedly what the thermostat said the temperature was in the house. He kept thinking his AC or heat or thermostat was faulty. Nope, it was him. I know I could have refused to go through this with him every day and simply give him blankets if he was cold or run a fan if he was hot, but I chose to do all I could to placate him because he was so touchy about everything. Every. Thing.

You could say Dad was fixated on his concern about being dropped, his finances, and the temperature in his house, and that would be right. But this was not the limit of his dementia-related focus. There were many fixations. And fixations on fixations. And urging me—relentlessly—to agree with what he was fixated on because how could I not see it his way?

He fixated on his new TV. His very old TV finally died in July, so I bought him a new one. This new nice flat screen TV had issues with the picture and the sound—that it didn't actually have. And we had to discuss all that was wrong over and over and over. And over. I had to purchase a sound bar so that he could hear the TV without his hearing aids, and he said that the sound quality was no good. It sounded just fine to me, and how could he determine sound quality without his hearing aids anyway? He thought the colors were off on the screen when the picture was really sharper and better than on his old projection TV. But this new TV was different, and in his world, different meant bad.

I learned the hard way that one of the most difficult dementia symptoms is that change is always bad, even beneficial change. For someone with dementia whose control is slipping away, change presents scary unknowns. In addition, the effects of dementia eliminate the ability to reason or rationalize; hence, what I saw with Dad was that he would hold tenaciously to a subject and be unwilling to let it go, and he would fixate on a variety of random things. In addition, the disease causes those with it to double down on conversation loops. In our case, it was often not that Dad forgot he had already discussed something with me, especially if it was a conversation he initiated. Instead, he seemed to need ongoing reassurance that I understood his concerns and agreed with them. All of these dementia-driven reactions must have been incredibly frustrating for Dad. They were maddening to me.

Another long-running fixation was on canned peaches, of all things. At his request, I bought him some, but they were not the right ones. This launched a diligent search for the peaches he just knew he had eaten in the past that were so good. Do you have any idea how many different kinds of canned peaches there are? And I don't mean just brands, but within the brands? I learned more than I ever wanted to know about canned peaches because I tried them all! It turned out the right ones did not exist. Sometimes, when I opened a new can, Dad would taste the peaches and say they were good. I would breathe a sigh of relief that I finally found the ones he said he remembered and wanted. But the next time he ate them, they had magically changed and weren't good at all. He would insist that they were not the same ones he ate yesterday. But they were. This inconsistency with knowing what he wanted showed itself in other ways too, and it was just frustration on top of frustration and more unpredictability in my daily life.

To compound the situation, Dad had hallucinations. This challenge began months before I began taking care of him. They started small and only happened occasionally, but increased in intensity and frequency as his dementia worsened. Instead of seeing things, as is typical, Dad's first hallucinations were smells. It was some time before I looked back and recognized this for what it was. He would tell me about a bad smell, and add that he called the city to complain, or he would inform me that there must be a plant in the area burning off bad chemicals because he could smell it.

Soon after I started caretaking for him, he began hallucinating about sounds. He informed me one morning that guys were working on the sewer all night, and all their noise had kept him awake. He also heard a song through the hum of his oxygen machine several times, and he could not understand why I didn't hear the hymn, too. It was "Sweet Hour of Prayer." Then later, he began seeing things. People in the house who were not there. A car wreck in the backyard. Bees flying all over inside the house. Rats behind the couch. Eventually, he hallucinated about people in the house who were there to steal his stuff. He insisted that they did, but of course, they didn't because they weren't there.

Awful.

ENDNOTE

1. Forgrave, Sarah. *Prayers of Hope for Caregivers.* Pgs. 19-21. Harvest House Publishers, 2019.

ENCOURAGEMENT FROM THE LORD

"How long, O Lord?
Will You forget me forever?
How long will You hide Your face from me?"

PSALM 13:1, NKJV

CHAPTER SEVEN

Desperation Before God

10/21/21 Journal Entry—

Looking Back ...

I gave myself away.

I lost all hope.

I lost myself.

I became entrapped, encapsulated, engulfed.

I lived in a completely different world with brand new rules that made no sense and constantly changed to become more and more nonsensical.

I lived with unpredictable, constant changes in what was and was not expected of me.

I experienced a darkness so deep that there was no perception at all.

Not even the tiniest pinprick of light anywhere.

Nothingness. Emptiness.

Utter aloneness.

Overwhelming fear always present.

The unknown loomed large and kept away any confidence in any decision-making effort in this completely foreign existence.

No rest.

No peace.

Some moments of comfort, but so fleeting, and sadly, always laced with dread.

Dread was a continual baseline infiltrating every breath.

A soul-deep longing for an end to this continual madness, and guilt for feeling that longing.

So many days when my goal was simply to survive the day.

So many days when I literally did not believe I would survive the day.

Some days when I didn't want to survive the day.

Desperation ...

I have experienced desperation before because I'm human, and I've lived some life. But I had never experienced it at this level. It was fierce and strong and pummeled me repeatedly every day for 112 days. And this was following the long period of Dad's decline leading up to the actual caregiving.

The enormity of what I was facing daily led to a desperation before God that included two-year-old, toddler-temper-tantrum, screaming, crying, beating-the-walls-in-the-shower meltdowns—and my screams were to God. Heart cries. Feral. No filters.

Almost a year after my dad passed away, I had a day when the old feelings surfaced in a flood of memories and pain. It all came into surprisingly sharp focus, so that I was able to write about it with a clearer understanding of just how desperate I was.

This desperation felt like ...

8/12/22 *Journal Entry—*

A vast, incomprehensible, impossibly rocky, dark, and steep path with shards of glass everywhere, and I'm barefooted. It's freezing, the wind is blowing and howling, and it's snowing, and I have no jacket, and my shirt is sleeveless, and I'm in shorts. I'm in a blizzard in the middle of winter, and there really is no path at all, no indication of which way is the way forward.

This is how I felt, and what makes this even worse is the huge gap between how I thought this would be and how it played out in a reality that taunted me. I visualized a path that might be a bit bumpy, but it would be springtime, with warm breezes and some flowers here and there. Ha. My future scenario vision was so sadly flawed that when it laid itself open, I was completely undone.

I'm fearful and careful and anxious anyway. All. The. Time. And I try to step cautiously so as to allow the giant of my fears to sleep. But that giant woke up, and he roared and knocked me flat. And I faced this alone. With no tools, and without even the right clothing for the occasion. No shoes—when I should have been dressed like an Eskimo, and I should have had my hiking boots on, you know, the ones I don't own.

Desperation.

When I began to see that all I could see was darkness and fear and defeat and depression and a longing for it all to end, I felt so guilty. This is not how a tough season is supposed to be responded to.

Why? Because I'm a deeply committed Christian. And deeply committed Christians are supposed to have faith and stand firm and not allow themselves to move away from all they know about how God is always good, and He knows what He's doing, and He's never surprised. Christians who are the real deal are supposed to "let go and let God," right?

But I was floundering and scrambling and struggling. And the reality of this daily life of caregiving kept knocking me down. I quickly reached the point that I just wanted to stay there on the ground in the dirt and stop fighting and give in. I wondered where God was because I saw no evidence that He was working toward making this all better. He was not even changing me to accept what was. He was not giving me the capacity to walk steadily through it with my head held high.

> Sometimes, from what our limited vision can see, God doesn't fix things at all.

Sometimes, God doesn't fix things like we think He should. And sometimes, from what our limited vision can see, He doesn't fix things at all.

I knew this, but somehow, I always thought when He didn't fix it, there would be an extra measure of *something* from Him to help navigate and work through whatever was going on. You know, like if you are hopelessly lost, but then you get periodic clues to help you find your way, or some sustenance to give you extra strength for the journey, or, I don't know, your favorite flower appears along the path to give you hope. Something … *anything* … extra that uplifts your mindset and spurs you on.

I don't know why I believed this because it's not spelled out in the Bible anywhere, but it became obvious during this season that this is what I expected. My expectation spoken from my heart to God looked like this: "You're not going to fix this? Fine. So that means I need You more, and I know You love me, so I should be able to feel You with me more, and I should experience otherworldly peace and confidence in the middle of all this." And then I would wait. And wait. Until I stopped expecting anything but more and more of this horrible new reality.

I did learn to look for and see glimpses of His presence in small ways that were huge to me because that's all I had.

While those instances felt wonderful, and they truly helped me survive, they provided only a brief respite. Before I knew it, I was right back in the middle of desperation. But you know what I learned as I began to look back after the season changed?

I learned that all my messy, mixed-up feelings were okay. Desperation, full-on everything out in the open emotions that I brought fiercely to God, fear and anger and frustration explosions, depression, defeat, and a gut-wrenching longing for the season to end ... all of it, it wasn't wrong.

How do I now know this? I did some praying, and some studying, and some listening to a sermon podcast from Dr. Tim Keller, who was a pastor I knew I could trust. And I learned. I learned that being desperate before God is okay because of two words: "Before God." I was desperate for sure, but I was desperate *before God.* I directed all my conflicting, chaotic, unpredictable, intense feelings to God. I addressed Him with all I was feeling.

I never stopped believing in God—not just believing *about* God, but *in* God. I believed in Him who created it all and holds everything together.[1] I just felt like He was choosing, for whatever reason, to allow me to feel very alone, and I was wrestling with that intensely.

One of Dr. Keller's sermons spoke directly to what I had experienced with Dad. I listened to it a few months after Dad passed away. I didn't search for it; it just appeared on my podcast app at the perfect time. Listening to it and soaking in its truths was so very helpful.

His sermon was part of a series on prayer, and this message, "Heman's Cry of Darkness,"[2] was based on Psalm 88:

> *O LORD, God of my salvation,*
> *I have cried out day and night before You.*
> *Let my prayer come before You;*
> *Incline Your ear to my cry.*
>
> *For my soul is full of troubles,*
> *And my life draws near to the grave.*
>
> *I am counted with those who go down to the pit;*
> *I am like a man who has no strength,*
> *Adrift among the dead,*
> *Like the slain who lie in the grave,*
> *Whom You remember no more,*
> *And who are cut off from Your hand.*
>
> *You have laid me in the lowest pit,*
> *In darkness, in the depths.*
> *Your wrath lies heavy upon me,*
> *And You have afflicted me with all Your waves. Selah*
> *You have put away my acquaintances far from me;*
> *You have made me an abomination to them;*
> *I am shut up, and I cannot get out;*
> *My eye wastes away because of affliction.*
>
> *LORD, I have called daily upon You;*
> *I have stretched out my hands to You.*
> *Will You work wonders for the dead?*

Shall the dead arise and praise You? Selah.
Shall Your lovingkindness be declared in the grave?
Or Your faithfulness in the place of destruction?
Shall Your wonders be known in the dark?
And Your righteousness in the land of forgetfulness?

But to You, I have cried out, O LORD,
And in the morning, my prayer comes before You.
LORD, why do You cast off my soul?
Why do You hide Your face from me?

I have been afflicted and ready to die from my youth;
I suffer Your terrors;
I am distraught.
Your fierce wrath has gone over me;
Your terrors have cut me off.

They came around me all day long like water;
They engulfed me altogether.
Loved one and friend, You have put far from me,
And my acquaintances into darkness.[3]

Dr. Keller's God-given insights in this sermon fully affirmed that I wasn't responding wrongly to all I went through. It was so comforting, like a healing balm, to have this affirmation that I did not respond to this situation wrongly.

Dr. Keller reminded me that most of us are naïve about the inevitability of suffering and tend to be shocked and ill-equipped when we face it. He quotes Martin Marty, a church theologian, who says this about Psalm 88: "Whoever tries to devise from Scripture a philosophy of life where everything always turns out right in the end will have to begin by tearing this page out of the Bible."

I used to have a simplistic view of what it meant to live as a Christian. Back then, it seemed logical to me that if you love God and pray and live right, life should always be good or have some level of good in hard times, like a silver lining. But the longer I live, the more I learn this is not always true. As Dr. Keller indicated in this sermon, sometimes you can do everything right and still have everything go wrong and stay that way for a long time. He further clarified that when everything goes wrong, there can be times when not only are you experiencing difficult circumstances, but at the same time, you are not experiencing much-needed peace and assurance from God. You feel alone, abandoned, and completely vulnerable to the grind of just trying to survive another day. This reality is what is described in this psalm. And a similar experience is the subject of David's prayer in Psalm 39, where he compares his life to being a vapor and lamenting how frail and weak he feels as he cries out, *"Hear my prayer, O LORD, and give ear to my cry; do not be silent at my tears; for I am a stranger with You, a sojourner as all my fathers were ..."*[4]

Many of the 150 psalms in the Bible are prayers amid intense suffering. Yet, most of these end on a hopeful note. Of all the psalms recorded, only Psalms 39 and 88 end in desperation:

"Look away from me, that I may smile again, before I depart and am no more!"[5]

"You have caused my beloved and my friend to shun me; my companions have become darkness."[6]

David, in Psalm 39, and Heman, in Psalm 88, bring all their emotions to God, unfiltered. These are not reverent prayers. They are not being respectful and choosing their words carefully. There is a complete lack of tempering their expressions to God with remembering who He is. Both prayers are examples of crying out in sheer desperation because they have nothing else left.

After sharing about the desperation of Heman and David, Dr. Keller asks an important question: "Why are these psalms in the Bible?"

He then shares a quote from Derek Kidner, who wrote a commentary on the Psalms. When discussing chapters 39 and 88, Kidner says, "The very presence of these prayers in Scripture are a witness to God's understanding. He knows how men speak when they are desperate."

Dr. Keller also discusses how Satan taunts God in the Book of Job, making it clear that he believes that Job only serves God because God gives him benefits.[7] One of the points Keller brings out here is that we often do this at the beginning of our walk with God. When tough times come, we point to all we are doing for God and ask Him why. But the truth is, we should be serving God because He is God, not looking to

Him to respond with rewards for our hard work. In these two psalms, the authors are praying with no expectation of any helpful response to their desperate cries for help.

But they pray anyway.

They keep bringing their responses to all that is going on in their lives before God. They do not turn away from God.

And that's key. Because in this choice of response, as Dr. Keller makes clear, Satan is defeated. Just like Job, these two psalmists chose to keep communicating with God about all they were experiencing in their struggle.

It amazes me that God chose to leave these two psalms and the Book of Job in the Bible. These Scriptures are such an encouragement to me. They ministered to me by showing that a high and completely holy God would allow, even encourage, us to be real with Him and not shrink back from expressing all we are feeling.

Praise God for His compassion, goodness, and love.

ENDNOTES

1   See Colossians 1:17.

2   This sermon was preached by Dr. Timothy Keller at Redeemer Presbyterian Church on November 4, 2007.

3   Psalm 88, NKJV.

4   Psalm 39:12-13, NKJV.

5   Psalm 39:13.

6   Psalm 88:18.

7   See Job 1:9-10; 2:4-5.

CHAPTER EIGHT

Worship And Hugs

I realized that if I wanted to be able to endure, something had to give. There had to be some positive change toward a healthier mindset, no matter how fleeting. God saw to this because He cares about every detail of our lives. He gave me small glimpses of hope—slight and brief, but nonetheless, very real.

This began with music, a lifelong love of mine.

God began bringing songs to my mind. And in a season where music, a mainstay all my life, was more than I could expend the energy for, worship songs and hymns just started playing in my head. I didn't have any desire to listen to music and had no energy to sing along, but God kept the songs coming, and I took this as a hug from Him. It felt as if He was graciously reminding me that I don't have to sing aloud or even listen to music playing to worship Him. And I felt a

> My longing to worship Him in the darkness made no sense, but God placed that yearning within me.

longing, an inexplicable need to worship, no matter what it looked like. My longing to worship Him in the darkness made no sense, but God placed that yearning within me.

Dr. Tony Evans said, "When joy has escaped you, it is time to worship. When life has crushed in on you, it is time to worship. When the devil has robbed you of your happiness, it is time to worship. When Satan has surrounded you or circumstances have surrounded you with things that bring you down, it is time to worship."[1]

I learned during this time exactly how what Dr. Evans said can be lived out when you feel you have nothing left to worship with. I had been crushed, my happiness robbed, and my circumstances brought me down. All that was true in this season, so it was time to worship.

For me, worship has always been most easily accessed through song. Of the songs that God brought to mind and I sang to Him in my head, many of them I had not thought of in years. God honored my worship, such as it was, singing without singing out loud. He heard my heart and accepted my feeble attempt to praise Him in the storm.

Dr. Evans' blog post goes on to say that worshipping when you don't feel like it will lift you up and bring you into the *"fullness of joy."*[2] This wasn't my story; I suppose because I had allowed the darkness to go so deep and become so heavy and overpowering. There was no room left for any other kind of fullness. Yet, there was a sense that God saw my effort and acknowledged that I was trying. And in a supernatural way, that hug from Him brought a small measure of comfort. That He would stoop low and really see me and give me any measure of comfort at all humbled me. It made me more mindful to keep doing it.

7/8/21 Journal Entry—

A shred of good within a tough day. This song started coming to mind last night. And I sang it in my head and heart. Lord, help me sing it obediently with Your joy and worship You today. Continually, in every lull, every rising of awful. Of dread. Of fear. Of sadness so deep there's no end.

The words of the worship song, "I Love You Lord"[3] ran through my head and stirred hope in my heart.

I don't have the energy or the motivation or desire to sing aloud. But I at least want to sing inside. I have not listened to any music or sung out loud in weeks. And that just shows the difference in this season because

> normally, I'm all about listening to music and singing along.
>
> Worship, that's where I start. Choose worship. Sing inside when I can't sing out loud because I just don't have it.

I made this an ongoing practice. I did it, especially in the mornings when I parked my vehicle in Dad's driveway right before I went inside his home for my day of caregiving with him. Standing at the door before I unlocked it and went inside to see what would greet me, I would pray for strength for whatever the day held, and I would sing a worship song in my head. Then, I tried to add more internal worship songs during the day when I could. And while it didn't change anything about what I was dealing with, it gave me a brief sense of a sort of normalcy, of groundedness, of choosing to remember who God is.

And then, there were little but helpful incidents, special "Hugs from Jesus."

Choosing to worship was in itself like a hug from Jesus. And there, in the middle of the awful, the desperation, the feeling of being all alone and completely isolated, the exhaustion so deep that I lacked the energy or desire to do anything except get through the day ... yes, in the middle of all that, God was ministering to me even though I didn't feel His presence. I did not feel He was providing His *"peace that passes all understanding."*[4] I did not have that kind of peace, but through this entire journey, He gave me beautiful, though brief, glimpses of Himself. Just enough to lift the darkness ever so slightly. I learned quickly to celebrate each glimpse because I knew I needed to hold fast to anything positive, no matter how seemingly small it was.

In my journal, I did my best to note these glimpses, these hugs from Jesus.

6/24/21 Journal Entry—

God worked a pure miracle today. I just knew after our long night last night that left both of us sleep-deprived today it would be horrible, a repeat of yesterday. But it wasn't like that. Dad was calm and not grouchy at all. No explanation, except this was a huge hug from Jesus. Much needed, much appreciated, so grateful.

7/18/21 Journal Entry—

A miracle. A break while Dad was napping that felt like a real break. Usually, when I take breaks, I'm just so exhausted. Breaks at home are relaxing, yes, but knowing I've got to go back to Dad's and dreading it ... that was not there this afternoon. It was so nice.

Thank You, Jesus, for giving me a real break that I could totally enjoy. I have not really enjoyed anything for a while. Thank You for the hug.

8/9/21 Journal Entry—

I got a Jesus hug. Cleaning out a cabinet today at Dad's, I came across Mom's old high school and college yearbooks—way cool. Excited about that. Thank You, Jesus, for something thrilling like this in the middle of the mess.

8/16/21 Journal Entry—

Good morning. I miraculously slept well last night when I just knew I wouldn't. That's a praise Jesus time. A hug from Jesus. Thank You, Lord, for good sleep because it does help. Never feel rested anymore—those days are gone, but a good night's sleep helps me deal with the day better because I'm coming at it not so exhausted.

8/18/21 Journal Entry—

Soooo surprisingly, truly, a miracle … today was soooo much better than yesterday. Even though I didn't sleep well again last night. There was this shift … I just felt more … centered, I don't know. Not as overwhelmed. I felt like it was going to be okay, eventually. Which was huge because I have been feeling—especially lately—like it will be just like my tough day yesterday forever. Exhausting, overwhelming, stressful, emotional, and hardly able to function almost … But today was Jesus hugging me and saying: "I'm here, you're not alone, I've got this, you can breathe." So I did. A little. Thank You, Jesus.

I began to learn how I needed to treasure every single positive thing. I understood that while every day won't have a hug from Jesus, there is always another one on the horizon. I wrote about this the day after the entry above:

8/19/21 Journal Entry—

I sailed yesterday. A nice breeze on the water. A reprieve. A breath. It was wonderful.

But there's no wind blowing this morning. The shift I embraced yesterday doesn't feel strong and positive and beautiful this morning.

But that's okay.

This is the ebb and flow of this season. Yesterday morning, I felt no wind either. But then, very gradually, a sweet, gentle breeze.

The day before yesterday, the wind blew me in the opposite direction into the fierce gale of a storm in the dark.

Ebb and flow.

And in the ebb and flow, this purposeful raising awareness of God's goodness helped me take notice of God and what He was doing to remind me how much He loved me. This was one of my lifelines that made a difference.

ENDNOTES

1   "Worship Is For You, Too" Blog Post by Tony Evans on The Urban Alternative. https://tonyevans.org/blog/.

2   See Psalm 16:11.

3   *I Love You Lord* by Laurie Klein © 1978 House of Mercy Music (Universal Music—Brentwood Benson Publishing).

4   See Philippians 4:7.

CHAPTER NINE

Cat Therapy

I believe God is mighty, holy, sovereign, and vast beyond anything I can imagine. But at the same time, I believe He is always working in every area of my life—from the daily mundane to the exciting and special. He orchestrates situations for my good that aren't huge life-altering moments but are important at the moment. And these wonderfully orchestrated scenarios can continue to prove how His unique design unfolds perfectly in my life. I believe this because I have experienced it in a wide variety of ways over the years. This is another way that I can see His incredible love for me.

One example culminated with my season of caregiving. This story began in 2018, but first, let me share the backstory to help you see the whole picture.

I had never owned a cat. I knew nothing about cats except I imagined that they were aloof and distant and not interactive and affectionate like dogs. Growing up, we always had dogs because my dad wasn't into cats at all. As an adult, I continued on with man's best friend for companionship. But after my last dog was put down in 2012, I decided I would not get another one until after I retired.

I have this wonderful girlfriend I've known for many years who has always been a cat person. After my dog died, she told me a few times that I should get a cat. I kept telling her I knew nothing about cats and didn't need a cat. So that was that. Until …

… September of 2018. One evening, she called me out of the blue to tell me that she worked with a cat rescue organization and had been volunteering at an animal shelter. She came across this cat she felt she should tell me about. Then she said the magic words—"He is so *calm* and *affectionate.*"

My heart responded with: *Hmmm. Calm and affectionate. Maybe I could use some of that in my life.* She made a point to tell me several times that there was no pressure.

"You don't have to decide right away," she encouraged, "and even if you make the five-hour drive to see the cat and choose to bring him home, rest assured that if he doesn't work out, I'll be glad to meet you halfway and you can give him back."

Her kind offer was tempting. My heart talked to me some more: *Calm and affectionate, no pressure, and if he doesn't work out, she will take him back.* I pondered it. And I added in the idea of how nice it would be to have a long-overdue visit with her and her husband—that sounded so enjoyable. How could I say no? So the next weekend, I drove there, met this sweet boy, loaded him up, and brought him home. He was a tuxedo cat, and I named him Oreo. (I know, original, right?) After the first few days of us getting used to each other, he proved to be exactly how she described him. As an added bonus, he was definitely a lap cat.

And here's where everything shifts from sweet and nice to what became significant and a part of the thread I held tightly to during caregiving. I learned pretty quickly that not only was Oreo calm, but he was calming—as in therapeutic— and I'm not kidding. I have known for years that people have "therapy animals" for various conditions. But I never dreamed I would have this experience. I had no idea that an animal could help me feel better, calmer, just by getting up in my lap and letting me pet him. But there it was, and it was much needed. I welcomed this when I got him in late 2018, and he served me well many times in 2019 and 2020 for a variety of reasons. But when 2021 came, and I became a caregiver to my dad, this therapeutic calming was especially essential. In fact, it was vital.

When I first got Oreo, I thought he would sleep in this nice, soft cat bed I got for him and placed in my bedroom. Nope. It became clear from the first night that his bedtime spot was in bed with me, and my idea was completely vetoed. I had sworn I would never let any pet sleep in bed with me again after the grief many years ago of losing a dog that actually passed away as I slept beside him. Dogs I had after this one were forbidden to do this, and because they were dogs, they complied. But Oreo steamrolled over my plans and substituted his. And I gave up. It turned out to be such a good thing. It was so sweet to have him in bed with me at night. I learned the comfort and joy of kitty snuggles. When I was caring for Dad, having that, even for a short time, on the nights I could be in my own bed was so helpful.

When Dad was napping and I could come home briefly for a break, I would sit in my recliner and Oreo would immediately get in my lap, curl up, and stay there purring while I petted him until he fell asleep. Petting him like this, some days even after he was sleeping, somehow helped my state of mind, however briefly. I can't explain it, but it was so real and so necessary. I hated when the time fell away far too soon, and it was already time to head back. I had to get him out of my lap and leave to return to my daily reality. But at least I had a small dose of comfort to carry back with me.

> God gave me the sweetest example of unconditional love—it had four paws and meowed ...

I had no idea that I needed a cat, but God knew. I had no idea that I needed cat therapy, but God knew. God gave me the sweetest example of unconditional love that had four paws and meowed, and it was like a soothing balm that went deep and touched hurting places inside.

Oreo was diagnosed with cancer in September of 2021. He started showing concerning symptoms, and a wonderful girlfriend took him to the vet for me because, by that time, I could not leave Dad hardly at all. After hearing the diagnosis, I prayed. I begged God not to take my beloved fur baby while I was still deep into all that went with caring for Dad. It was just too much to fathom. I prayed that Oreo would not continue having the symptoms and pain that brought about the vet visit. I prayed that he would live for at least a while longer without suffering. In God's perfect demonstration of answered prayer, Oreo immediately stopped showing pain symptoms and did very well until December, two months after my dad died. I made the difficult decision to have him put down on December 4, 2021. I have a framed picture of him, his pawprint, and some clippings of his fur on display. He was a beautiful gift from God to me, a rare gift that kept on giving throughout the three years I had him.

This story has a nice postscript. Having Oreo showed me that I'm a cat person, and I just never knew this fact. So now I have another cat. I got her four months after Oreo passed, and her name is Kiki. She literally chose me. As soon as I sat down at the shelter to see if another cat I had my eye on would get into my lap, Kiki bounded up and stayed there, purring like she belonged there—and well, I couldn't say no to that! She's quite different from Oreo in looks and personality, but she is perfect for me at this time in my life. She's not what I would call calm. Sweet and affectionate, yes. Calm? No. Kiki is shy and fearful of anything or anyone new. After over a year, she has mellowed quite a bit but still sometimes runs and hides. God's timing is perfect. I'm retired now and have much more time to spend with her than I ever did with Oreo. I can work with her, play with her, and encourage her whenever she needs to feel secure. She's also a great therapy cat, but sometimes we give each other therapy.

God is good all the time, and He cares about every detail. Thank You, God.

I'm so glad my dear friend thought to reach out to me that day in 2018, trying to find a wonderful cat a home. Neither of us had any idea how important that phone call would prove to be as the story it initiated unfolded in my life.

CHAPTER TEN

Caring For a Caregiver

I'll be honest; I have struggled—a lot—with how to share this part of my story. I've prayed about it, seeking guidance from God. And I've even considered whether I should share this at all.

I know how I felt about the things I'll be describing here, but I didn't want to show any negativity about any of the sincere, caring responses to the struggles I was walking through. I didn't want to share that any response was anything but helpful. I know that every single dear friend I interacted with during this journey wanted the best for me. They all intended to help in ways they thought might lessen the heavy burden I was carrying, and I appreciate everyone's efforts. I really do. I am grateful and so blessed to have so many people who care deeply about me and my well-being.

That said, I feel a deep desire to share some things I learned in an effort to help someone else. These are things I plan to put into practice in the future when I come alongside someone struggling with caring for an aging parent (or parents) or any other loved one. I want others to know what kind of response was like a glimpse of light in the darkness to me, as well as what just didn't work that way for me. That means I feel the need to share what was genuinely helpful, but also what was ... not so much.

So what was the "not so much"?

A response that fell into this category went something like this: "I completely understand. I've been where you are."

When someone you love is going through a hard situation, and maybe you've had a similar experience, it feels automatic to want to let them know you completely understand. I get it. You want them to feel like they are not alone. And knowing you are not the only one to endure a particular challenge can be very comforting. But sometimes, "I've been where you are" diminishes what you are enduring. Without meaning to, it can reduce the high hurdles you encounter to a common experience. And that leaves you feeling misunderstood.

Some basics are similar in every caregiving experience, especially for elderly parents. So, another person who cared for their aging parent does have some understanding that others do not. A certain level of empathy exists among those who care for aging parents or other relatives. But there are also some differences in each specific situation. Every family dynamic is unique. Variables that come into play include the health of the relationship before the caregiving began, whether the decline is mental or physical or both, other life demands that coincide, financial details, logistics, the health and wellness of the one providing the care, and more. No "one experience sums it all up" tips and tricks exist. There are no universal answers.

Yes, every caregiving experience, at its core, is unique. Yet, I fall into a family dynamic category that is not the norm. I know there are others like me out there somewhere, which is one of the reasons for this book. My story has its own twist. I'm single. I'm an only child. Why is that so important?

These details added an entirely distinctive level to everything about my journey. Without a spouse or sibling for support or relief, additional layers of difficulty, stress, dread, and hardship were added to my burden. These facts created a slightly different angle to the path I walked. It made my path just different enough that when others expressed to me that they completely understood, I knew without a doubt that they didn't, not fully. They couldn't. My path looked different from theirs because it was different.

Other than God, I was completely alone. Doing it all. All the responsibility was mine alone, with no one to discuss options with who knew my dad as I did. I had no sibling to bounce things off of and ask for feedback. I also had no spouse to support me when they saw how I was being affected. I do have a wonderful extended family, and I'm blessed by all of them, but they did not see Dad as I saw him. They did not have the insight of immediate family. The only immediate family was me.

Am I being too picky here? Too sensitive? Maybe, but this is how I felt, and I want to be transparent and share what I learned that I want to apply in the future in reaching out to others who find themselves caring for their loved ones as they age. In a way, I feel like I sound plaintive, like I am a spoiled child feeling sorry for myself. But that was my positioning for this season. I was a single only child, and that did make a tough time tougher. That was my reality. Honestly, the only person who completely understood what I was going through was God. In a way, that is true for everyone. *"Each heart knows its own bitterness, and no one else can share its joy."*[1]

> The only person who completely understood what I was going through was God.

Something I take from this is that I want to be mindful of others and simply be there for them. I want to ask what they need. Pray for them. Check on them. Ask if it would be helpful to share what worked for me and share it if they want to know. Refrain from anything further than sharing my experience and allow them to use the information in any way that might be beneficial to them. I want to listen to them. Dignity is extended when you allow someone to share what they are going through and just listen. Being heard is comforting. I want to affirm the feelings they share. Being affirmed is a bit of peace in a tumultuous time.

What did I find most helpful?

- People who were simply present.

  In a way, they were similar to Job's friends at the beginning of his story.[2] They just sat with me (figuratively because I was isolated), and they listened (via text), and they loved me. These people reached out to check on me often. Then they listened and loved some more. Some asked if they could share their caregiving experiences. Others asked if they could point me to some resources that might be helpful. And they listened and loved some more.

  They offered to pray for me and reminded me often that they were praying. One beautiful friend reached out with inspirational art or scriptures periodically. What she sent always came at the right time to briefly lift the heaviness.

- Affirmation.

  I talked to one dear friend about how I felt so alone yet felt guilty for feeling alone because I knew God was with me, and I was not living like I knew this. She lovingly affirmed me. Rather than try to refute my perspective, she said, "Lauri, you literally are alone. You are doing this on your own with no physical person to walk through it with you. Having no one to listen to you or give feedback on decision options must be so hard. I am sorry for how alone in this you are."

  Her affirmation was hugely helpful. I felt seen.

- My safe place.

  I have four very close friends who were a lifeline. They were safe and constant and chose to stand for me when I couldn't. They stood and held me up where my faith had waned and my hope had vanished. We were in a group text together. One day, I sent them a text to vent my frustration. I was mortified as soon as I hit send. I immediately sent another text apologizing, telling them I was okay and just having a bad day. I didn't want them worrying about me or thinking ill of my dad. I got immediate responses, and they made some things very clear to me:

  They were already worried about me, and that would continue.

  This group text place was a completely safe place. They loved me unconditionally and encouraged me to unload here. They knew I had a very real need to vent to someone, and they were up for it and wanted me to do it.

  So I did. Vent. Often. And just knowing they chose to hear me and love me all the way through was so precious and treasured. They were a literal lifeline.

I am a work in progress on loving others well. It's easy for me to get wrapped up in myself and what I feel or want or need instead of thinking more about the other person. However, I want to apply everything I learned during my caregiving journey and use it to be more loving and caring to others.

I want to see them more as Jesus sees them. Specifically, I want to apply what I learned to be a beacon of the love of Jesus to others within the storm of caregiving.

I hope sharing the responses I experienced from the friends I thank God for helps you know more about showing love to another in a caregiving journey.

ENDNOTES

1   Proverbs 14:10, NIV.

2   See Job 2:13.

ENCOURAGEMENT FROM THE LORD

"Praise be to the God and Father of our Lord Jesus Christ, the Father of compassion and the God of all comfort, who comforts us in all our troubles, so that we can comfort those in any trouble with the comfort we ourselves receive from God."

2 CORINTHIANS 1:3-4, NIV

CHAPTER ELEVEN

Crisis Care

By the last few weeks of Dad's life, I felt like I belonged in a caricature of the old saying, "At the end of my rope." Or, there I was, the cute kitty in the picture barely hanging onto a tree branch with the caption, "Hang in there!" Except nothing about this was humorous or lighthearted. Hanging on was becoming increasingly harder. The rope was unraveling.

Dad grew more and more impatient and frustrated. His angry outbursts were part of the daily nightmare that was my life. They were a given. I just continued to do the best I could. I lived in the nightmare and was now at the point where I saw no way out. As weird as this may sound, I can totally relate to the dismal attitude of those who feel like whatever negatively impactful experience they have in life is all there is. You can reach a place where your entire focus is just trying to get through each day in any way you can. You have nothing left to think of anything else. You are locked in survival mode.

But then, one day, he went so far over the top that I immediately texted his hospice nurse. I was officially at the very end of the rope, and I didn't know if I could keep hanging on. I knew it was time to reach out and let the nurse know what was happening and hope she could do something to help. Actually, I know now that it was past time to do this.

A new conversation began toward the end. Dad did not realize he was at home. He would ask: "When are we going home?" sometimes several times a day. Each time, I would tell him he was home, and he would let it go. But on October 1, he asked me this question again, and when I responded that he was at home, he became extremely frustrated, paranoid, and accusatory. His ongoing angry outbursts had several levels of intensity, and this one was off the charts. He accused me of lying to him about being at home when instead, what I was really doing was keeping him from going home. He said, "I don't know what you're doing, but I know you're lying to me. I know for sure that I'm not really at home. I don't know why, but you don't want me to go home. I won't stand for this! I will walk home if I have to. I demand that you take me home!"

I wasn't worried about him walking home as he had threatened because he could not even sit up without getting dizzy. But I was worried about him refusing to trust me and being so belligerent and angry. I responded with the most patient tone I could muster, "Dad, I am not lying to you. You truly are at home. I'm sorry you don't believe me." Then I went out to the garage on the pretense of getting clothes out of the dryer, and I texted his hospice nurse, who, thankfully, responded immediately that she would come by soon to check on him.

While waiting for her to arrive, Dad needed me to do something else for him, and I was taking care of that when she showed up. I believe that God set this up because, for the first time, someone else got to see what I was enduring on a daily basis. The nurse witnessed one of his angry outbursts as she watched us interact. This one was less intense, but still, he was yelling at me and upset that I could not satisfy him when he did not know what he wanted. She checked his vitals and told me, "I recommend we begin Crisis Care with your dad. This can help to alleviate his agitation and make him more comfortable."

I stood looking at her, unsure if I had heard right. It sounded like a way to help him that might also be helpful to me. But I had no hope left, so I waited for more explanation before I responded.

The nurse looked me in the eyes and, with compassion in her voice, she said, "Crisis Care provides nurses to be with your dad 24/7 in shifts. Your dad would be medicated continually to keep him calm. Are you okay with that?"

I did not need to think about how to answer this question. The rope I was hanging onto kept separating, and the pieces kept getting more frayed, and my arms were so tired. My answer was an immediate, resounding, and relieved, "Yes." *Oh, yes, please!* A desperate yes. A grateful yes.

Crisis Care comes into play when the hospice company determines that the patient needs constant monitoring and medication to make them comfortable. It is not considered until the patient is in severe pain or is severely agitated. The hospice company I used contracted with another company that sent LVNs to the home to administer this level of care.

So, while I knew the basics of what Crisis Care was, I didn't know everything about it. I thought it was typically for patients in great pain. I really didn't understand what was meant by "severe agitation." I just assumed it was much more than what I was experiencing with Dad, like if someone was extremely combative or physically violent. I had no idea that Dad's level of agitation qualified him for this care.

Praise God, it did.

After discussing Crisis Care with me, the hospice nurse talked to Dad directly, very kindly. She placed her hand gently on his arm and said, "I know you are miserable. I know you are really uncomfortable. We have a way to help you. We can provide you with nurses around the clock to give you medication so that you feel much better."

Dad did not argue with her, which was a shock to me. He simply said, "Okay." After the nurse left, Dad had his last lucid moment. He asked me, "Does this mean I will be medicated until I die?"

I swallowed hard and said, "Yes, Dad. It does. We know you are suffering, and this is a way to alleviate that. I don't want you to suffer anymore."

His response surprised me. My daddy's last coherent words to me were, "Bring me my razor."

And then, he shaved his whiskers.

Looking back now, that makes me smile. My dad was probably the most practical person ever, and I think his last words were the perfect fit for the personality God gave him. No, it was not the movie ending I had envisioned, where his last words would have been expressing love and appreciation. But God showed me in other ways that Dad expressed his love for me deeply until the very end.

A new journey started on the afternoon of October 1, 2021. The hospice nurse administered Dad's first dose of medication to start calming him before she left. The first Crisis Care LVN arrived that evening for the night shift.

The specialty of Crisis Care nursing requires more expertise than I realized. Before I watched this process unfold with Dad, I thought Crisis Care nurses would administer medications to keep him sedated, which in my mind equated with unconsciousness. As in completely out of it, like a deep sleep. I could not have been more wrong. I have no medical expertise, but I learned a lot from what I witnessed. My new understanding is that Crisis Care means medications are given to help the patient relax and rest, but not to the point of losing consciousness completely. When done correctly, it's a very delicate and compassionate dance—an intricate art form. It is highly complex and individualized care. The goal is to keep the patient in a state of peaceful calm, while still conscious enough to understand vocal expression and respond to questions.

I watched this dance play out beautifully starting the next day, which began the last two days of Dad's life here on earth. The dance was incredibly and wonderfully performed by the nurse who arrived that morning for the day shift, a nurse that I can only describe as angelic. And I mean that. She was an angel sent from heaven.

Her presence at the end meant I did not have to manage his final moments alone. The value of that gift cannot be measured. A gentle, reassuring, ongoing hug from Jesus.

When done correctly,
Crisis Care is a very delicate
and compassionate dance—
an intricate art form.

CHAPTER TWELVE

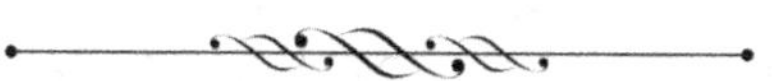

Angelic Nursing

I have always had a high level of respect and appreciation for nurses. All nurses. But then, sometimes, special ones touch your life with such love that you never forget them. I've been blessed greatly in the past by nurses who took their job of knowledgeably caring for others seriously and added compassion and lots of grace.

Before October 2, 2021, I had been blessed twice by what I call angelic nursing.

The first time, I was a young brand new mom still in the hospital after having my son late the night before. I had family and friends visiting all day long starting the morning after I had him because it was Saturday. My "Angel of Rest" nurse saw me—*really saw me*—as I walked by the nurse's station when I finally had a break from nonstop visitors. She gently but firmly ordered me to gather what I needed and go to an unused patient room that had a jacuzzi. She added in a no-nonsense yet kind tone that I was to stay there until I felt better. I remember sitting in the tub sobbing. My tears expressed overwhelming new mom fears and exhaustion. But there was also a sense of incredible relief—good tears—because the pulsating jets and warm water felt wonderful, softly ministering to my body, mind, and soul.

The second angelic nurse was my "Angel of Crisis." I encountered her when I was transferred to her rehab center from the hospital after a car wreck. God chose her to check me in, and she noticed an issue with the catheter. She left the room to get equipment to investigate further but literally came running back in when I started screaming in pain from what turned out to be a catheter blockage. She was so tender and gentle as she resolved the issue and checked on me several times that night. After this crisis was over, she made a point to check on me at least once a day for the whole two weeks I was there, even when my room was not with the rooms she was assigned for her shift.

These two nurses showed me such comforting love and care, far above and beyond what was expected.

I was then blessed by angelic nursing a third time, by my "Angel of Caretaking." She arrived at 7:30 a.m. on Saturday, October 2. I had not had a good night. At all. The first Crisis Care nurse who worked the night shift was part of the reason, and that's a long story I won't go into. But because my experience with her was far less than stellar, I was not expecting anything better and really dreading what the new day shift nurse might be like. I remember watching out the front window for her to arrive, wondering if she would bring an even more horrible experience than I had already endured. I saw her drive up and went to the front door to let her in. And suddenly, with no warning, the heavy, dread-filled atmosphere lifted. All she did was introduce herself. She simply said, "Good morning, I'm Nurse Regina." But there was an immediate and beautiful connection to me expressed in her whole demeanor and those few words of introduction. It was an amazing gift—a Holy Spirit connection. Praise God—I just knew, deep within, that I could breathe now ... for the first time in what felt like so long.

And that supernatural knowledge I felt deep within proved to be so right. She came in like a calming breeze. A breath of fresh air. It was like God whispered to me, "She's got this; you don't have to worry about anything. She's Mine, and she works for Me." Oh, the relief in this knowledge—I can't tell you how amazing it felt. After being "the one" for so long who had to decide everything and take care of all Dad's needs the best I could, she came with not only expertise born of education and 20+ years of experience in caregiving for dying patients, but also with an incredible amount of love and compassion for her patients and their caregivers. She interacted with my dad like he was the reason she was there—because he was. Whenever she interacted with him, even though he did not appear to be conscious, she would talk to him just as she would converse with anyone. She introduced herself each time and called him "Mr. Walter." She then would let him know what she was about to do, something like, "Mr. Walter, I'm going to give you another dose of this medication now; I need you to open your mouth so I can get it to you quickly and help you feel better." And he would comply. Then, she would let him know when she was done and ask him if he needed anything else to make him more comfortable. His responses were unintelligible to me but not to her. If he moved or tried to express himself verbally when she was not by his side, she would approach the bed and then run through a series of questions. She always determined what he needed and lovingly worked to provide it for him.

On this, her first day with him, he was in a lot of pain. She knew this because he would start moving around a lot only a little while after each dose of medication. And he would scrunch up his forehead, which she said was a sign of pain. She kept on patiently working with him, checking in with hospice, gradually increasing medication, and trying different combinations until he was resting well. It was like a graceful ballet, where each complex move added more depth of kindness. And she involved me every step of the way. She told me everything she was doing and why and patiently answered all my questions.

And then she took this incredible care to the next level. She did something I will never forget. I was running around the house late in the afternoon, doing all the usual daily stuff. By this time, Dad was resting well, and she was sitting and making notes. She stopped me in my tracks with these incredibly kind words, "I am not only here for your dad. I am here for you, too. Please tell me something I can do to help you."

What???

I was incredulous, completely shocked, and taken aback by this because it just never occurred to me that this would happen. I was by now very accustomed to doing everything myself all the time. It was already so beyond anything I could imagine that someone was finally here that I knew without a doubt I could completely trust to take wonderful care of my daddy. I never thought she would even consider wanting to help me, too. It blew me away. It was not a huge gesture, but it was hugely kind. An extra affirming and calming gift from God. A hug from Jesus that was not letting up. He continued to draw me closer in His arms.

Yes, she was an angel. In a nurse's uniform. Much like the other two I described earlier. But in this season, I needed her so much more than I needed the others. She was a balm to my overwrought, exhausted soul. I will never forget her.

Thank you, Nurse Regina. You were truly the hands and feet of Jesus to me.

ENCOURAGEMENT FROM THE LORD

"I sought the Lord,
and He answered me;
He delivered me
from all my fears."

PSALM 34:4, NIV

CHAPTER THIRTEEN

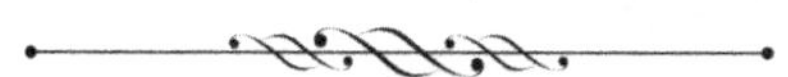

The New Beginning

10/03/21 Journal Entry—

It is 10:12 p.m. Dad passed away around 2:30 this afternoon. What a day. I feel such sweet relief that he is no longer struggling and suffering.

Yes, the very first emotion I felt upon Dad's passing was an incredible, huge, uplifting relief. An indescribably heavy weight lifted, and I thanked God again for Regina, the angelic Crisis Care nurse. God chose her to be with us on his last day of life here.

Soon after Nurse Regina arrived for her shift on this morning, I left briefly to go home, shower, and change clothes. I was only gone for a few minutes. When I returned, I learned that

Dad's respirations dropped from 18 to 8 as soon as I left. A hospice nurse had arrived to check on him while I was gone, and both nurses agreed that he had chosen this time when I was not there to begin transitioning to end his life here and begin it in his eternal home. Regina said, "Ms. Lauri, even though your dad is not obviously conscious, he is aware of your presence. He also knows your voice and understands what you say. He knew you had left, and he chose this time to turn the corner toward dying to spare you the pain of being present for this choice. I've seen this happen many times."

I didn't respond. Instead, I chose to allow the enormity of what she said to go deep as I embraced the bittersweetness of what this meant. This realization was a final and very special hug from Jesus. This final act of kindness showed me that underneath it all, my daddy was still there. Beneath the dementia. Beneath the gradual but escalating faster and faster alteration of his personality. Beneath the intense and crazy fixations and hallucinations and confusion and frustrations and anger and paranoia. Yes, he was still there, still loving me as much as he could and still thinking of me and giving me the best he could give me. He was still there, choosing to wait until I was not present to begin the end of his life with me. Trying to spare me pain.

It brought me a measure of comfort.

Before Dad died that day, I talked to him two different times, telling him that I would be fine, my son would be fine, and it was time for him to let go and leave us and go enjoy the best reunion ever with Mom and my sisters, Janet and Nancy, in Heaven. I told him to give them all big hugs from me. After I did this the second time, it was not long before he moved on to his new beginning.

I know that I gave this season my all. ALL. While I definitely did not do everything right, I know that I did the absolute best I could do to honor Dad. Now that it was over, I found that I was glad I did this. I will never wonder if I should have done more.

The relief that I felt immediately after Dad died stayed with me. It was accompanied by sadness, but I did not experience deep grief. I was not distraught. As time went on and the expected tears and days filled with sadness did not come, I wondered what was wrong with me that I was not grieving as a "normal" person should when a loved one dies. I expressed my concerns and questions with a few trusted friends, and they all told me the same thing without communicating with each other. They confirmed for me that I started grieving the loss of my dad a long time ago. Because dementia began taking him away from me gradually, then faster and faster, I had been saying goodbye to him in stages all along the way. My grief intensified during the time I was his caregiver.

Because dementia began taking him away from me gradually, then faster and faster, I had been saying goodbye to him in stages all along the way.

When he died, it was just a final chapter in a long, hard grief process, and there was comfort in the closure. He was no longer fighting all he could not understand, no longer angry, no longer miserable. He was now at peace, so I could also be at peace.

I believe that God left me clueless about all I was getting into when I chose this caregiver journey because had I had even the slightest glimpse into what it would look like, I would have run screaming in the other direction. And I'm absolutely sure that had I known just how bad it would get, especially in the last few weeks, I would have done just about anything to avoid experiencing it.

But God wanted me here, in this season, in the impossibly hard and scary and sad and frustrating and overwhelming and depressing and oppressing. He wanted me here to show me how what you can't possibly do gets done when He chooses to intervene miraculously. I didn't see any of that in the thick of it, but I can see it now.

Many things about this season were continually torturous. But the hardest part was the aloneness that permeated almost every moment of every day. I despaired that God was even there for me. I felt abandoned. I felt like God checked out and said, "You're on your own, My child. Just do the best you can, and I might watch you sometimes from way over here." But God didn't watch. And He was not a long distance away. I wasn't just a tiny spec on the horizon that He might focus on occasionally. No. Instead, He held my hand and was right by my side the entire time. He never left me. He never forsook me. He lovingly walked with me through the valley of the shadow. I could not see or feel Him, but that does not make it any less true.

The fact that I survived it is truly a miracle. The fact that I did not end up sick or in the hospital is another miracle. During this season, I truly believed two things quite regularly: 1) I was utterly alone, and 2) I literally would not survive.

And there were times I wasn't sure I wanted to survive. I seriously felt that dying was an inviting option to consider. I did not want to take my own life, but if I died, I didn't see that as a bad thing. Because then it would be over. And I wanted it to be over, which meant either I wanted Dad to die, or I wanted to die. That sounds terrible, but it was my reality.

I can look back now and know that God saw. God understood. God was all over this all the way through. I panicked and looked everywhere and saw only all the impossible. I couldn't see Him, and that was terrifying. It appeared that He was not anywhere.

> I see God now— everywhere.

But I see Him now. Everywhere. His timing. His provision. His love. His understanding. His patience. His compassion. His love for Dad. His love for me.

I wish I could have lived through this with deep, unwavering faith. But I didn't. Yet, I have realized that in my distorted view of God's truth, He still chose to work through the shattered lens I was using. I'm grateful. I was His instrument in this, as flawed as I was, and I was used to honor Dad's wishes. And that could have only occurred because God kept me—held me fast—secured me—surrounded me—though I felt nothing but the violent storm raging.

In God's timing, soon after this journey ended, I began working on what I felt God was calling me to do. A deep longing began when this journey started and had sat dormant but no less intense within me ... now that longing came forth and flowed into words on a page.

And what you hold in your hands is the result of that longing.

I hope this book has been at least a little helpful, shining a glimmer of light into your darkness.

And I wish I sat across from you and could impart to you just how much I care about what you're experiencing and how much I want to offer all the encouragement your heart can hold.

Caregiving, no matter the specifics, is tough. For me, in some ways, it felt like my previous world exploded. But in the messy fallout that remained, I learned that there is a beauty that will shine forth when you can look back. You will see that your choice to do all you can to care for someone you love is a choice that costs more than you can imagine—but it truly is worth it.

You will survive, even when you believe that you won't. And you will embrace your life again.

Darkness builds faith and strength and light. These are all waiting to be released. You will behold that beauty. And it will be incredible.

Your light will be even more brilliant after the darkness recedes.

ENCOURAGEMENT FROM THE LORD

*"He put a new song in my mouth,
a song of praise to our God."*

PSALM 40:3A

ABOUT THE AUTHOR

Lauri is a grateful recipient of the love of Jesus. He leads her on ongoing adventures of the soul as she continues digging deeper to gain knowledge and understanding of the incomprehensible grace and "God-ness" of God. Her passion for writing is inborn and she is honored to share it as a ministry tool to encourage others.

This book is the result of a clear calling from God. Lauri is qualified to write about the many facets of caregiving because she experienced all of them with her dad in the last months of his life. God placed a deep longing within her to reach out to others with her story. She brings a real, raw, unfiltered testimony and offers it fully to the reader. She chooses to make herself vulnerable because it's that important to reach those who need assurance that they are not alone in their struggles and the accompanying myriad of emotions that make up any caregiving journey. She also wants to testify about the love of God, who does not turn away from desperation and painful unrehearsed heart cries, but responds with tender compassion every time, even when it is not evident until later.

Lauri is honored that you would take the time to read her story, and she hopes that it brings encouragement and hope.